Leg Ulcer Treatment Revolution

Professor Mark S Whiteley

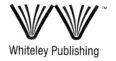

Whiteley Publishing

Published by Whiteley Publishing Ltd
First paperback edition 2018
ISBN 978-1-908586-05-6

The information in this book has been supplied by the author
and has been published by the publisher in good faith.

Contents

Leg ulcer treatment revolution

Prof Mark S Whiteley

Introduction

Patients who have venous leg ulcers know exactly what ulcers are. However, many people who are unaffected by leg ulcers are not really sure what they look like. For those who do not know what venous ulcers are, they can best be described as an "open sore" in the lower leg. It is an area where the skin has broken down, revealing the underlying tissue.

Not surprisingly, these open sores weep fluid, can get infected, can smell and can be painful. Traditionally, doctors and nurses treat venous leg ulcers by putting dressings on the open sores, and by applying pressure on the area with compression bandages. This is the way that leg ulcers have been treated for over 100 years and, unfortunately, is still the way most doctors and nurses have been taught how to deal with them.

Since the mid-1980's, new technologies and research has shown that this is often not the optimal treatment. We now understand that most venous leg ulcers can be cured, saving the country or state in which the patient lives, huge amounts of money in dressings and nursing care, getting the patient back to mobility and a normal life, and freeing carers or family from the responsibilities of looking after a patient with a chronic problem.

There cannot be any question that curing a venous leg ulcer is a good thing. Whether you look at this financially, morally, from the view-point of society, or the quality-of-life of the patient, their family or their carers, there really are no arguments against trying to cure leg ulcers permanently.

So why don't we?

I am sure there are many reasons why doctors and nurses have not changed their practices to cure the large numbers of patients with venous leg ulcers that can be cured permanently. A great many companies earn money from dressings and bandages. Many doctors, nurses and other healthcare workers work with outdated protocols and do not question them as many busy professionals do not keep up with the latest research or guidelines. There is always a resistance to any change, and this is nowhere more evident than in medicine and nursing. There may be other factors as well.

The point of this simple book is not to point the finger of blame at anyone.

I have spent the time to write this book merely to educate anyone, patient or professional, who is interested in what we now know about venous leg ulcers and wants to cure those that can be cured.

Hopefully, some patients will read this and will take action, with the result that their chronic, relapsing leg ulcer disappears forever, giving them a new lease of life.

Hopefully, some carers or family members of patients with venous leg ulcers will read this and take action on behalf of the person that they care for, to achieve the same benefit for the patient.

Hopefully, some doctors, nurses and other healthcare workers will read this and realise that if they change their protocols and follow the new research and guidelines, they will be able to achieve a permanent cure for a substantial proportion of their patients, releasing resources for those that are incurable.

I have tried to make this book short and simple, and have added lots of diagrams, hoping that it is easy to read and understand.

I sincerely hope that this book will result in a great many patients with venous leg ulcers finding out that they are curable and finding the cure that they need.

August 2018

Typical cases of a venous leg ulcers that were cured with endovenous surgery

with a cautionary medico-legal warning

Of the hundreds of cases of leg ulcers that I have treated and cured over the years, I have included two cases as they are highly representative of the problems that patients with leg ulcers face at the current time.

Over the years I have assessed and treated patients with venous leg ulcers at virtually every age of adult life. The youngest was 19 years old. Leg ulcers become more common with advancing years, however, many people are shocked at just how many people have venous leg ulcers in their 40's and 50's.

Several of the adult patients that I have seen, came to me because they had lost their jobs. They had been dismissed because they had needed to have their legs dressed twice a week, and the smell of the ulcer became difficult for people around them at work.

Recently, we treated and cured James Turpin, a man in his 30's who had developed his venous leg ulcer at age 24. Since the age of 12, his nick-name at school had been "snake boy", because of the huge varicose veins that ran down his legs. Since developing the ulcer, he had seen multiple doctors and nurses, and had been in constant dressings and compression since. He had been a waiter and then a restaurant manager – but had been unable to work due the ulcer.

Worse still, some of the doctors that he had seen over the years had refused to believe that such a young man could develop a venous leg ulcer. As such he had been given several rare, and incorrect, diagnoses. He ended up being given steroids which resulted in him having 5 fractures in his spine, and also a course of chemotherapy!

As it turned out, he had a simple venous leg ulcer secondary to his venous reflux and stasis. He underwent endovenous surgery under local anaesthetic (endovenous laser and TRLOP), followed some weeks later by ultrasound guided foam sclerotherapy, with the result that his ulcer healed and has never come back.

His post-operative course was difficult with the sudden change of activity and venous blood flow, and he did develop a DVT early in his recovery. However, this did not cause much of a set-back and, as we would expect, within 3-6 months his ulcer had completely disappeared as had his DVT.

For the first time since he was 24, he is out of compression bandaging, and can start building a life for himself. He has taken up running and cycling, but now must put the wasted years behind him as he enters the job market, with good legs for the first time.

We have many such stories, all showing the huge impact that leg ulcers have on patients and their families. However, the following case is more typical in terms of age and wasted time and resources due to the current way leg ulcers are managed.

This story is also about a lady called Janet Cassie. You will see her photographs on the cover of this book.

Janet came to see me in October 2016. She was 68 years old and was generally very well. However, she had been suffering with a right sided venous leg ulcer for four years. Over those four years, her district nurses had tried many different dressings and many different forms of compression. Sometimes the ulcer appeared to be improving, sometimes it appeared to be worsening, but it never healed.

Janet needed to have a left hip replacement and was getting

increasing amounts of pain and immobility from her hip. However, her orthopaedic surgeon refused to operate on her hip with an open ulcer, due to the increased risks of infection of the new joint.

In desperation, Janet sought specialist advice. I saw her in October and our team performed a venous duplex ultrasound scan. This showed that she had venous reflux in her great saphenous vein (the vein which runs from ankle to groin just under the skin) and that she had eight incompetent perforators. In addition, she had dilated veins under the ulcer, which are "stasis veins". Most importantly, and like most of the patients we see with venous leg ulcers, her deep veins were normal.

There were only a couple of small visible varicose veins on the surface and, because of that, she had always been told that her ulcer was not due to varicose veins. However, although she did not show great numbers of varicose veins on the surface, she did have underlying venous reflux in the same veins that usually show as varicose veins. It is because of this confusion that I introduced the term "hidden varicose veins" almost 10 years ago.

In December 2016 I performed endovenous laser ablation under local anaesthetic to close her incompetent great saphenous vein and TRLOP closure of the eight perforators using endovenous laser. This was all done at one procedure under local anaesthetic. Janet walked in to the procedure and walked out of the clinic 2 hours afterwards without any complications.

In February 2017, her ulcer was healing well, and she underwent ultrasound guided foam sclerotherapy to destroy her stasis veins.

In April 2017, the ulcer was almost completely healed and in May it was completely cured. She did not need any compression at all and had returned to a completely normal life. She has not needed any compression since.

Later that summer she was able to have her left hip replacement.

The cost of her treatment, including investigations, was £5,450. With Janet's permission we performed a freedom of information request to look through her notes and found that in the preceding four years, over £25,000 had been spent by her GP practice on dressings, compression and medication. This did not include nursing time, travel nor the time of various consultants who had seen her previously.

Janet felt very aggrieved that she had lost four years of her life to a chronic condition that she had been told was not curable, which then turned out to be curable. She threatened to sue her family doctor and district nurse. I offered to go and give an educational talk to the practice saying that if they learnt from the experience, perhaps that would help her come to terms with the situation.

In autumn 2017 I went to the practice and gave a talk, explaining everything that is in this book and how, by using these principles, we had cured Janet so quickly after so much time and money had been spent in not curing her.

At the end of the talk I was thanked for my time. I was told that there would be no plans to change the pathway of investigation or treatment for any other patients with leg ulcers in the practice, as the doctors and nurses were comfortable with their guidelines! The fact that the NICE guidelines had changed did not influence them.

To me, it is obvious that if we were to change our way of investigating and treating patients with venous leg ulcers, we would end up with many advantages for both patients and society. Patients would be freed from disability. Families and carers would be able to return to normal life or to do other work. Nurses and doctors who specialise in wound care would be able to concentrate on patients who had incurable leg ulcers and wounds. As shown by Janet, curing venous leg ulcers would end up saving huge amounts of money for those who fund healthcare.

It would appear to me that there is no downside to taking on the lessons outlined in this book and illustrated by Janet's case. This is why I am passionate to spread the understanding of venous leg ulcers, to help empower patients and their carers to find a cure for their venous leg ulcers, and to educate those doctors and nurses who are willing to listen.

On-going medico-legal position

As this book is going to press, I have had a letter from Janet and her solicitors. Their expert advice is that the family doctors looking after Janet failed in their duty of care, by not referring her for a cure of her venous leg ulcers when they saw her in 2015, as the NICE CG 168 guidelines had been produced in July 2013. In addition, the nurses looking after her had also failed in their professional duty in reporting that the doctors had failed in their duty.

As this news has only just arrived, I cannot say whether any action will follow nor what the outcome will be if it does. However, it is clear that there is a revolution occurring in the treatment of venous leg ulcers – and not before time!

Mark S Whiteley August 2018

Chapter 1

Leg ulcers - heal or cure?

As described in the introduction, a leg ulcer is often thought of by the public as an "open sore".

Thinking about this more medically, we must think about what covers the body. Most of our body and certainly our legs are covered with skin. When we break the skin, we have a wound. A wound usually heals. When a break in the skin does not heal and remains open, it is called an "ulcer" (Figure 1).

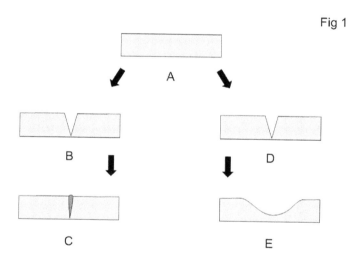

Fig 1

Figure 1: Simple diagram to show the difference between healing normal tissue with a scar, and a cut forming an ulcer. A represents a cross-section of normal skin. B shows a cut which then heals normally with a scab followed by a scar – C. However, if there is an underlying problem interfering with the normal healing process, the same cut D fails to heal. This then becomes a chronic wound or an ulcer – E.

In medical terms, any long-term break in the surface layer of the body is called an ulcer. You may well have had a mouth ulcer where the inner surface of your cheek, lip or tongue has broken down exposing the underlying tissue. As you know this can be sore and it leaks fluid. You can also get ulcers in your stomach or intestine. Most people have heard of a "stomach ulcer" and know that this can perforate the bowel or bleed.

The aim of treatment for any ulcer is to try to allow the body to grow normal tissue back over the open sore. Of course, this results in the ulcer disappearing. When this happens, is this healing the ulcer or curing it?

You may think that there is no difference in these two words. Indeed, in many circumstances you can probably use them interchangeably.

However, when we talk about leg ulcers it becomes far more important to think about the difference between these two words. In fact, it is the difference between these two words that has caused me to set up The Leg Ulcer Charity, write this book and has massive ramifications for patients, their families and carers as well as for the finance of healthcare in any country or state.

Healing versus cure

When nurses or doctors apply dressings to a leg ulcer and compress it, they are aiming to heal the leg ulcer that they can see. They dress and compress for weeks, months or even years to try to encourage skin to grow back over the open sore and to "heal it". When the skin completely covers the ulcer, they feel that it has been "healed". To them, this represents a success.

The problem is, they haven't done the one thing that is actually needed to heal the ulcer and to stop it from coming back again. They haven't identified the underlying cause of why the leg ulcer started in the first place, nor have they corrected it. Therefore, not surprisingly, the same ulcer will come back again in the majority of patients in the future. When a leg ulcer is "healed" by dressings and bandaging alone, this is only a temporary healing and not a permanent cure.

Conversely, when an ulcer is cured, it means that the underlying cause of the ulcer has been identified, the cause has been treated and, because of this treatment, the ulcer heals and remains healed permanently - i.e. is cured.

Underlying causes of wounds and ulcers

When we think of the usual sorts of wounds that we get on our bodies or limbs, we know the natural way that they heal. If, for instance, someone gets a graze on their knee after falling onto hard ground, then we know that it will form a scab and that it will heal (Figure 2). The reason that it heals is that the underlying cause for the graze was trauma - i.e. falling over and scraping the skin on the ground. As soon as we stand up, the underlying cause has been removed and the healing process starts. This healing process is called "inflammation", and we will come onto this later.

In patients with venous leg ulcers, it is a completely different story. Some people with venous leg ulcers will remember a traumatic event that started the "wound" such as a cat scratch, or banging the leg. However, in normal limbs, such minor trauma would heal. In patients who develop leg ulcers, there is an underlying cause which interferes with the healing. The normal healing process does not occur, the skin does not cover the open wound and so an ulcer develops as an open sore.

The usual underlying cause is a disturbance of the venous system, although sometimes it might be due to an insufficiency of the arteries. Causes other than venous or arterial problems are rare.

Most people who develop venous leg ulcers already had signs

Fig 2

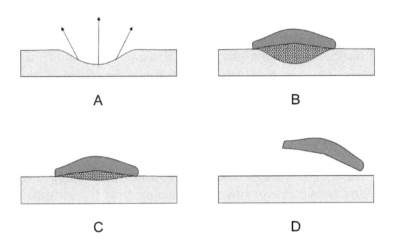

Figure 2: If an open wound occurs, such as a graze, or an ulcer where the underlying cause has been treated, then normal wound healing can take place. An open wound – A – oozes plasma. This is the water and protein from the blood without any blood cells in it. If this is allowed to dry – B – the protein forms a scab, trapping sterile plasma underneath it. This sterile plasma contains nutrients and growth hormones, the perfect environment for the tissue to re-grow – C. When the tissue has filled in any deficit and skin has grown to cover the wound, the scab falls off – D – leaving a perfectly healed wound.

of an underlying problem before they suffered the trauma and developed the leg ulcer. Such signs might be varicose veins of the affected leg, a red discolouration of the skin of the lower leg, a brown or brown and white discolouration of the skin of the lower leg or a hardening of the skin and tissue of the lower leg (Figure 3). These are all warning signs that there is an underlying vein problem which is already causing inflammation and damage of the skin in the lower leg. It only takes minor trauma to break this inflamed skin and hence start the process that results in non-healing and a venous leg ulcer.

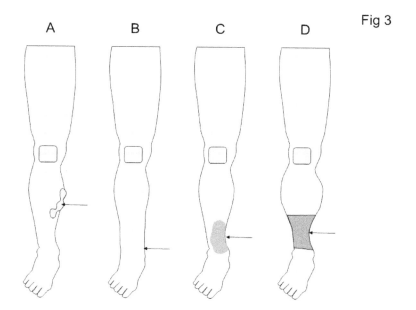

Figure 3: Common signs of varicose veins or "hidden varicose veins" causing tissue and skin damage heading towards leg ulcers. A – varicose veins. B – swollen ankle (often normal in the morning but swells as day goes on, especially in hot weather or if sitting for long periods of time). C – the "gaiter area" where venous skin changes usually show first: venous eczema (red and itchy), lipodermatosclerosis (skin and underlying tissue gets harder in this area and often become shiny and a yellow colour), hemosiderin (brown), atrophie blanche (brown with white patches – close to ulceration). D – "Champagne bottle leg" where the tissue in the lower leg is so inflamed it gets very tight, causing the calf to bulge.

No matter what doctors, nurses or other healthcare professionals try to do to that wound, it will become an ulcer if they fail to deal with the underlying problem that is causing the inflammation in the skin and tissues in the area. Once formed, the ulcer will either remain unhealed, or will heal temporarily, only to come back again in the future, unless the underlying cause of the ulcer has been identified and treated successfully. Dressings and compression bandaging alone do not address the underlying cause of the ulcer nor fix it. Therefore, although they may cause a temporary healing, they will not lead to a permanent cure.

Scabs and wound dressings

Most venous leg ulcers leak fluid to a greater or lesser extent, at some time. Such leaking fluid can be a great problem for patients as well as for doctors, nurses and other healthcare professionals looking after ulcer patients. Much of the nursing literature about how to treat venous leg ulcers relates to removing scabs and then dealing with the large amounts of fluid that leak out of the ulcer. Although we will come back to this area later, it is probably good to start thinking about this very early on in this book.

In all areas of medicine, it is useful to correlate something you know and understand that happens in one situation and think about the same problem in a different situation. You can then see if your understanding fits both scenarios. If it does not, then your understanding might be wrong, or you may well have been taught something incorrectly.

Let's go back to thinking about a graze on the knee. Most of us have had such a graze at least once, often as a child. As we showed in Figure 2, when we graze ourselves, the skin is removed forming an acute wound which we call a "graze". We usually clean this, may put a temporary plaster on it, to keep it clean, but one way or the other we let a scab form knowing that it will heal under the scab.

Why does it heal?

What is actually happening in this situation is that the fluid leaking from the wound is plasma. Plasma is the fluid part of the blood but without the blood cells. It is full of protein.

The way that humans heal a surface wound like a graze is that the water in this fluid evaporates away, allowing the protein to form a "cap" over the graze. At first this is soft and mushy and

24

may be mistaken for "infection". However, with further drying, the protein goes very hard and becomes a scab.

As children we know that when a scab comes off, there is good, new pink skin underneath. The reason for this healthy skin regeneration is because of the scab. As the plasma leaks out of the wound, it pushes any bacteria or debris out of the wound. As the plasma dries and forms a scab, the scab forms a protective cover, stopping any new infection getting into the wound.

Underneath the scab, the proteins in the plasma include a high proportion of growth factors. Growth factors are proteins that stimulate the skin cells to reproduce, forming new skin under the scab. When the skin has completely regenerated, the scab falls off revealing the new pink healthy skin.

So why do our wound care experts forget this when it comes to treating venous leg ulcers?

When the body develops a venous leg ulcer, it follows the same strategy to try and cure this open sore. However, the usual treatment from doctors, nurses and healthcare professionals is to put a dressing on the ulcer that stops a scab forming! Indeed, nurses are usually taught to remove scabs from ulcers. It is common practice to remove all scabs before dressing a venous leg ulcer, and then to put a new dressing over the ulcer in its place. The dressing is used to try to keep infection out and keep the area under the dressing perfect for healing – exactly the same functions that the scab was performing naturally and for free!

Many of these dressings are costly and have several beneficial claims made about them. However, it does not take a genius to realise that we have taken nature's own perfect dressing, that has formed at exactly the right time of the healing process and is made of exactly the right substances for the individual patient and taught our nursing staff to remove it and replace it with something else to try to exactly mimic it. Of course, this keeps nurses busy and provides good profits for companies making popular dressings.

A scab, when formed, stops the fluid leaking onto the surrounding skin. If the scab is removed and replaced with dressings, the fluid can leak onto the surrounding skin. This can cause maceration (the skin goes wrinkly and then white) and inflammation. This often looks like infection as the skin initially goes bright red and is often very sore, before turning white and then dying and breaking down. The death of the surrounding skin results in the ulcer increasing in size.

Another major problem to consider is the amount of protein escaping from the patient in this plasma. If the fluid is allowed to keep on escaping from the ulcer, then the patient is losing all of the protein that the fluid contains. Many patients with leg ulcers do not have a high-protein diet and not surprisingly, if blood samples are taken from these patients, they are often found to have very low protein levels. Low protein levels in a patient can lead to increased swelling of the limbs which worsens the condition of the lower legs. It also reduces the healing powers of the body, as the immune system needs lots of proteins to make antibodies and white blood cells that fight infection and help with healing.

We will talk about this later in the book. However, you should already be getting the message that allowing air to get to a venous leg ulcer, and to allow a scab to form, will often stop a venous leg ulcer getting bigger and will start the healing process better than most dressings.

However, we can't just say to everyone "stop dressing leg ulcers and allow then to form scabs", as we have to get the leg ulcer into a position that it can heal before starting to use this sort of strategy. This means that we have to sort out the underlying causes of the leg ulcer and correct them first. Just letting air get to a venous leg ulcer and letting a scab form on it will not cure it, unless we have already fixed everything else and the leg ulcer is ready to heal permanently and be cured.

In the next chapter we will talk about the underlying causes of leg ulcers, and how to find out which one is responsible for any particular leg ulcer.

Chapter 2

Underlying causes of leg ulcers

As we have already discussed, a wound anywhere on the skin will heal unless there is an underlying problem either preventing the healing process or causing the wound in the first place. When a wound is in the lower leg and it does not heal, it becomes an open sore called a leg ulcer. So, what are the reasons that the skin in the lower leg might not heal?

In order to heal, the skin needs to have a good blood supply. This means that there needs to be a good supply of blood with oxygen and nutrients in it. This comes from the arteries. In addition, waste products such as carbon dioxide and urea need to be removed and taken away from the area so that they do not accumulate in the tissues underlying the skin. This removal of waste products is performed by the veins.

Arterial blood flows in the arteries and is full of oxygen and nutrients. It is under high pressure from the heart and always flows forwards unless the arteries are blocked.

Venous blood sits in the veins and is full of carbon dioxide and waste products. It is under very low pressure. It will not flow out of the legs unless it is pumped out by movement, or the legs are compressed from outside with stockings, bandages or pumps, or finally the legs are elevated so the blood flows out of the legs and back to the heart by gravity.

The commonest causes of leg ulcers are venous causes, followed by arterial causes.

There are also other causes of leg ulcers, but these are really quite uncommon compared to venous causes. Many people talk about diabetes as a cause of leg ulceration, and there are also other causes such as rheumatoid, lymphoedema, infection, and vasculitis. For the purposes of this book, we can ignore most of these as they are rare. Diabetes does not cause leg ulcers by itself, but only if the diabetes has affected the arteries or very small arteries called arterioles, that supply oxygen and nutrients to the skin. As such diabetes is not so much the cause of leg ulcers by itself but it might be associated with other causes, particularly arterial insufficiency.

The majority of leg ulcers (somewhere between 70 to 90% of all leg ulcers) are venous. Fortunately, it is these leg ulcers that are the easiest to cure permanently.

Therefore, we are now going to concentrate on venous leg ulcers for a while.

Venous leg ulcers

Venous leg ulcers almost always occur in the lower leg around the ankle and up to the calf, usually on the inner aspect of the leg (see Figure 4). They can sometimes occur on the front, back or outer aspect of the lower leg. Uncommonly they can affect the foot just under the ankles or even onto the top of the foot. However, venous conditions do not cause ulcers on the end of the foot or around the toes.

A venous leg ulcer is often irregular in shape.

They are usually associated with one or more of the conditions mentioned in the last chapter and illustrated in Figure 3 - varicose veins, red stains, brown stains, hardness or swelling of the lower legs.

We will discuss the causes of venous leg ulcers next, and once we have done so, you will understand the following points. Venous leg ulcers improve when the leg is elevated, particularly if the ankle is higher than the heart and the leg has been elevated for some time. Indeed, one of the simplest tests to tell if a leg ulcer

Fig 4

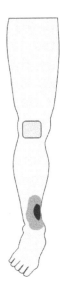

Figure 4: Typical position of a venous leg ulcer, although they may occur elsewhere on the lower leg or foot.

is venous is to admit the patient to hospital, give them blood thinning agents to stop them from getting clots in the veins, and then keep them in bed 24 hours a day for five days with the bed tipped so that the ankles are higher than the heart. If it is a venous leg ulcer, and all dressings are removed and kept off the ulcer, allowing air to get to the surface to form scabs, the ulcer will show great signs of healing and the surrounding skin will start to look healthier.

As most people can't be admitted to hospital for such a time, we have to rely on other manoeuvres. If a patient improves with compression, such as wearing compression bandaging or compression stockings, then it is usually a venous leg ulcer. Such improvement with compression helps us to diagnose that the ulcer is venous, but it is important to understand that this improvement with compression is not a cure. Compression merely improves the ulcer temporarily whilst it is in place. This will be explained further as we go through the book.

Venous leg ulcers are often more tender when the leg is allowed to hang down to the floor when sitting. This is worsened if there is no movement in the leg and the blood is allowed to pool in the veins around the ankles by the action of gravity.

Tests for venous leg ulcers will be discussed in more detail later, but the gold standard test for venous leg ulcers is a venous duplex ultrasound scan. This is NOT a "Doppler", which is a very simple test to measure the blood pressure in the arteries at the ankles.

Arterial leg ulcers

The other main sort of leg ulcer is an arterial ulcer. An arterial leg ulcer is caused by the arteries being blocked or narrowed. This results in insufficient blood getting to the lower leg and toes, to keep the tissue alive and healthy.

Arterial leg ulcers usually occur on the outer part of the lower leg or on the foot and toes. Arterial ulcers are often "punched out" with a very regular edge. They are usually very painful.

Arterial ulcers get worse when the leg is elevated as the very low blood pressure in the blocked or narrowed arteries cannot overcome gravity. It is common for people with arterial leg ulcers to wake up with pain in their toes or feet in the middle of the night and have to hang the leg out of bed, or to get out of bed and sit in a chair. This manoeuvre raises the heart above the feet and allows gravity to help blood flow around blocked or narrowed arteries in the legs.

As arterial leg ulcers are caused by low blood pressure in the arteries after the blood has had to get around blocked or narrowed arteries in the legs, compression on arterial ulcers will make them worse, as will elevation of the leg. Hence arterial leg ulcers get more painful with compression or on elevation of the leg.

The cure for arterial leg ulcers is to improve the blood supply which usually means a bypass graft or opening the arteries with a balloon or stent.

The first test for arterial leg ulcers is to measure the blood pressure at the ankle with a Doppler. It is amazing that although only 10% of leg ulcers are arterial, doctors, nurses and healthcare professionals are trained to assess leg ulcers with a Doppler. However, once they find that the Doppler pressure is normal, most fail to proceed to the specialist test that is needed to diagnose the far more common venous leg ulcers - a venous duplex ultrasound scan.

Chapter 3

Causes of venous leg ulcers

As we discussed in the previous chapter, the circulation to the lower leg needs arterial blood to take oxygen and nutrients down the leg, and venous blood to take carbon dioxide and nutrients away.

If venous blood is allowed to stay in the veins in the legs, it sets up a very unhealthy pooling of stagnant blood in the veins. This stagnant pooling is medically called "stasis".

Many doctors, nurses and healthcare professionals probably do not think much about the pooling of blood, nor consider that it might be particularly damaging for the patient. However, more and more research is showing that this sort of stagnant blood or "stasis" blood is actually very irritant to the veins and tissues in the lower leg. When the tissues get irritated, they get inflamed. When tissue gets inflamed over a very long time, it starts getting damaged.

So why does stasis blood cause irritation and inflammation?

Blood is not a fluid. The fluid part of blood is called plasma. Plasma is water containing lots of electrolytes and proteins in solution. There are cells suspended in the plasma. The combination of these cells and the plasma mixed together is blood. Most of the cells in blood are called red blood cells. These red blood cells are full of haemoglobin, the red pigment in blood. The haemoglobin carries the oxygen in the blood.

In addition to red blood cells, there are white blood cells. White blood cells are used to fight infection. Some make antibodies and some attack bacteria, viruses and cells that are misbehaving in the body. Finally, there are platelets. These are small fragments of cells that are used in clotting.

All of the cells in the blood are living and as such need oxygen and nutrients themselves. In stagnant blood sitting in stasis veins in the lower leg, the blood cells continue to live, using up any oxygen and nutrients left in the surrounding stagnant blood. This results in increasing levels of carbon dioxide and waste products in the venous blood lying within the stasis veins.

One of the essential features of why this stagnant blood is so irritant to the veins and surrounding tissues is the build-up of carbon dioxide within it. Many people do not realise but when carbon dioxide dissolves in water, it forms an acid called carbonic acid (Figure 5).

Fig 5

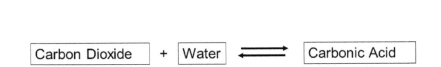

Figure 5: Carbon dioxide gas, when it dissolves in water, becomes acidic – an acid called "carbonic acid".

When the arterial blood flows through the tissues and then collects in the veins, it is already low in oxygen and high in carbon dioxide. Hence venous blood is already quite acidic. In addition to the acidity, there are also other waste products in the venous blood that make this situation worse. If this blood is allowed to stay stagnant in the veins, this acidic blood causes irritation and inflammation of the vein walls and surrounding tissues in the lower leg. Also, the longer the blood stays in the veins, the worse the situation gets. This is due to the continued build-up of more carbon-dioxide and waste products (Figure 6).

Fig 6

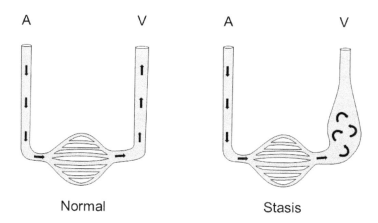

Figure 6: A diagram showing how venous stasis can interfere with capillary supply to the tissues. A is the arterial blood flowing into the capillary network in some tissue in the leg. V is the venous blood flowing out of the capillary bed. In stasis, the veins have dilated, disrupting the smooth flow through the capillaries.

Therefore, it becomes very obvious that the simplest way to improve a venous ulcer is to get this stagnant blood out of these "stasis" veins in the lower leg and back to the heart. Once it gets back to the right side of the heart, the venous blood is pumped to the lungs where the carbon dioxide is removed and is replaced by oxygen. The other waste products get removed by the liver and kidneys. This is how the body gets rid of the waste products from venous blood and converts it back to new arterial blood, full of oxygen and nutrients to keep the cells alive.

This simple understanding will help you make sense of some of the things that doctors and nurses already do to help patients with venous leg ulcers.

For instance, we know that this stagnant blood in the "stasis" veins causes inflammation in the veins and tissues in the lower leg, which over the long term leads to worsening damage and venous leg ulcers. Hence, when we elevate the leg above the level of the heart, this blood flows back to the right heart by the effect of gravity, and so reduces the amount of inflammation in the lower leg. This explains why venous leg ulcers start to heal when affected legs are elevated.

Also, as the stasis veins are dilated and full of venous blood, it is not surprising that when we put compression bandaging or compression stockings on the lower leg, this squashes these stasis veins. Squashing these reduces the amount of stagnant blood in the lower leg, and by reducing this, reduces the amount of inflammation.

Therefore, by this simple understanding of only one part of the venous cause of leg ulcers, we can already see why some of the traditional ways to treat venous leg ulcers – elevation and compression - seem to help in the short term.

However, neither of these have actually made any permanent changes to the stasis veins nor to the lower legs. They are merely temporary measures to reduce the amount of stagnant blood in the "stasis veins". As soon as the affected leg is not elevated any more, or the compression is removed, the original stasis veins will open up again and the patient is back to square one.

Therefore, what we really need to know is what causes this blood to become stagnant and collect in the "stasis veins". Or put another way, to include all the causes of venous disease, what causes inflammation in the veins of the lower leg?

Three main causes of venous leg ulcers

There are three main venous causes of inflammation occurring in the veins of the lower leg and surrounding tissues. Each of these three causes, if left untreated, will go on to cause inflammation of the veins, damage to the surrounding tissues and venous leg ulcers.

These are:

- venous stasis
- venous reflux
- venous obstruction

Venous stasis

We have already discussed venous stasis (or stagnation) above but have only thought of it so far as an isolated problem in the lower leg.

Venous stasis often coexists with venous reflux or obstruction. To understand the links between venous stasis and venous reflux or venous obstruction, we must think about the veins and how they usually function in a living person. We will come on to discuss how venous stasis occurs as a result of venous reflux or obstruction later, but we have to add one more situation where venous stasis occurs alone before we can continue on to consider the other two situations.

It is possible for venous stasis to occur in patients with normal veins. Indeed, although not common, some patients with venous leg ulcers have them totally due to venous stasis alone with no other cause.

In these patients, venous stasis occurs because of lack of movement of the leg. As we noted previously, there is very little pressure in the blood in the veins in the lower leg at rest. When someone lies down flat, there is just enough pressure in the venous blood for it to flow back to the heart. However, when you sit or stand up, there is not enough pressure to push the blood out of the veins in the foot and lower leg, to get it back to the heart (Figure 7).

Therefore, for venous blood to flow back to the heart from the foot or lower leg, it has to be pumped. This pumping occurs by movement of the foot or leg. When a person stands up and puts

Fig 7

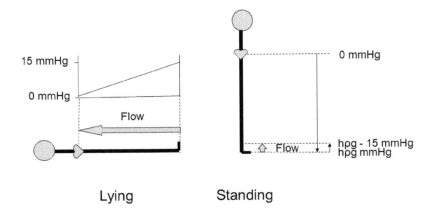

15 mmHg

0 mmHg

Flow

Lying

0 mmHg

Flow

hpg - 15 mmHg
hpg mmHg

Standing

Figure 7: A diagram showing how different positions affects the venous pressure and hence flow back from the ankles. When lying flat, the pressure of the blood as it comes out of the capillaries and enters the veins is 15 mmHg (15 millimeters of Mercury). This is just enough to get the blood back to the heart which is at 0 mmHg. However, when standing, the pressure of the column of venous blood from the ankle to the heart is much larger than this pressure. This means that when standing, the venous blood only gets to just above the ankle bone. Technically the pressure is hpg – where h = the height of the column of blood, p = the density of the blood and g = the acceleration due to gravity. (Reproduced with consent from: "Understanding Venous Reflux: The Cause of Varicose Veins and Venous Leg Ulcers by Mark Whiteley)

weight onto their foot, the foot flattens, and blood gets pumped from the foot into veins in their calf muscle. When they wiggle their ankle, or start walking forwards, the calf muscle contracts, pumping blood further up the leg and into veins in the thigh. When the leg is lifted, the thigh muscles coordinate with the others to continue the venous pump action, forcing more venous blood out of the leg and back to the heart.

When walking, all of these pumps coordinate giving a maximum return of venous blood to the heart from the legs. This is why walking is such a good exercise for veins (Figure 8).

Fig 8

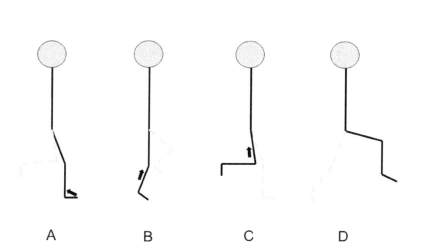

A   B   C   D

Figure 8: Diagram showing how walking pumps the venous blood back to the heart. A – when the foot is first placed on the ground, and the weight is transferred onto it, the foot flattens, squashing and stretching the veins in the foot and pumping the venous blood into the calf (the "foot pump"). B – as the weight shifts forwards, the calf is contracted to propel the body forwards, and the foot is used to "toe off". This contraction of the calf muscle pumps the venous blood upwards to the thigh ("calf pump"). C – As the leg is lifted off of the ground, the thigh muscles contract, pumping blood into the pelvic veins ("thigh pump"). D – as the leg swings forwards ready to take another step, the muscles relax and the blood starts to reflux. This causes the valves in the veins to close, stopping the venous blood from refluxing (in the normal person). (Reproduced with consent from: "Understanding Venous Reflux: The Cause of Varicose Veins and Venous Leg Ulcers by Mark Whiteley)

However, if you are sitting in a chair for a very long time without moving, blood starts pooling in your lower leg, becoming stagnant. If you are on an aeroplane, and there is a low oxygen level in the atmosphere due to the altitude and partial pressurisation of the cabin, this pooling of the blood can result in the blood clotting. This clot is called a deep vein thrombosis (DVT). This is why you are advised to wiggle your feet, walk about the cabin or to wear a travel sock (compression stocking) when flying long distances.

Although this problem of venous stasis due to lack of movement is highlighted for travellers, it is not highlighted in many other people who suffer from this condition. For instance, if you visit homes for older people where they sit for long periods of time watching television or doing other sedentary activities, it is very common for these people to have swollen ankles, skin changes around the ankles or even venous leg ulcers, just the same as those shown in Figure 3. In these patients, there is often no venous reflux, and these problems are merely due to the lack of movement of the ankles and feet. In this situation, these skin changes or leg ulcers are quite correctly called "venous stasis changes" or "venous stasis ulcers", if the other veins in the leg are completely normal.

However, in the majority of people who suffer from venous leg ulcers or show skin changes, the stasis is secondary to venous reflux. As such, these terms should not really be used unless venous reflux has been excluded by the patient having a venous duplex ultrasound scan.

Venous reflux

Venous reflux is the name given to the condition where venous blood falls or flows the wrong way through a vein, away from the heart. In its simplest form, it is due to the valves within the veins not working. I will explain this more fully as we go on. However, it is important to note that venous reflux is very common in the population, affecting somewhere between 30-40% of adults in the western world. The problems of venous reflux range from leg varicose veins to venous leg ulcers, varicocele (varicose veins around the testicle in a male), varicose veins around the vagina or vulva in females, pelvic congestion syndrome, haemorrhoids (piles) and an increasing number of other conditions.

Although it appears to be quite simple at first glance, venous reflux can actually get quite complex. It is because it is complex that so few doctors who treat varicose veins get good results, as few doctors specialise only in venous research and treatments. If only the simple forms of venous reflux are understood, it is not surprising that patients only get simple treatments, often for quite complex problems. Hence the high failure rate and why so many people get their varicose veins back after treatment. It is also why doctors shy away from treating venous leg ulcers, as many do not get good results for the same reasons.

I am going to discuss venous reflux as it relates to venous leg ulcers more fully in the next chapter. However, if you get interested in venous reflux and want to know more about it after reading that chapter, I have written a book called "Understanding Venous Reflux - the cause of varicose veins and venous leg ulcers" that is widely available online and all good book sellers can order it, if they do not have it in stock.

Venous obstruction

Venous obstruction is the name given to a significant narrowing or a blockage of a major vein, which reduces the blood flow through it. You might think that a blockage in a vein would stop blood flowing through it completely. However, when a vein blocks, in almost every case, tiny veins that flow around the blocked section of the vein start to dilate, acting as a partial bypass. These veins are called "collaterals". This makes a blockage act more like a severe narrowing than a complete blockage.

For many years, doctors and nurses didn't bother investigating any patient with venous leg ulcers if they had had a deep vein thrombosis (DVT) in the past. Such patients were told that there was nothing that could be done for them because their deep veins had been "damaged". As such they were consigned to a life of compression bandaging and compression stockings.

Research over the last decade or two has shown this to be completely wrong. Most patients who have a leg ulcer and a history of a DVT, have normal deep veins when tested.

This is because a single DVT, that is recognised early and treated aggressively with anticoagulation therapy, often resolves without any damage to the deep veins. Therefore, a great many patients who have been told that there is "nothing that can be done for them" actually only have venous reflux, and could be cured easily.

Some patients have had multiple DVTs, or a DVT that was so severe and lasted so long, that it caused permanent scarring or damage of the deep veins. When associated with a swollen leg, with discolouration and leg ulcers, this is called "post-thrombotic syndrome" (PTS). Again, such patients have been told in the past that because of the deep vein damage, there is "nothing that can be done" and once again these patients are consigned to a life of compression bandaging or stockings.

However, research has shown that such patients often have a narrowing or blockage that can now be opened up with a balloon, and the vein kept open with a stent. This has been so successful that many people who have been virtually crippled with swollen legs and long term recurrent leg ulcers have got back to completely normal lives following treatment with stents. Most often, patients have to have anticoagulation which nowadays means a tablet every day. However, this is a small price to pay for cured leg ulcers, a leg that has come back to normal size and the ability to walk normally again.

We are going to talk about venous obstruction in more detail in a later chapter.

For now, we are going to concentrate on the most common cause of venous leg ulcers, venous reflux.

Chapter 4

Venous reflux, and how reflux causes leg ulcers

As mentioned before in this book, blood in the veins should flow back to the heart. Also, we have seen that venous blood is full of carbon dioxide and waste products. It has to get back to the heart against gravity, so that it can be circulated through the lungs, kidneys and liver to get rid of the carbon dioxide and waste products. It can then pick up more oxygen and nutrients to be recirculated as arterial blood again.

Also, as pointed out before, venous blood is at low pressure and only flows back to the heart by itself when we are lying down (Figure 7). As soon as we sit up or stand up, the heart is higher than the ankles and venous blood cannot flow naturally back to the heart without help.

This is where we need the venous pump, to pump the venous blood back from the legs to the heart.

However, before we talk any more about flow in the veins, we really ought to know a bit more about the veins in the leg, and how they are arranged. It is going to be important to have a basic understanding of the main veins so that you can understand some of the important facts later in this book. Hence, I will make this as simple as possible,

Veins in the leg - deep veins, superficial veins and perforator veins

In the leg, there are many different sorts of veins. In the simplest form, these can be divided into two groups, deep and superficial (Figure 9). For any doctors and nurses who come on my courses

44

or read any of my other papers or books, it is important to know that the superficial system is split into two and so there are actually three groups, or layers, of veins. However, for the purposes of this book this detail is not required.

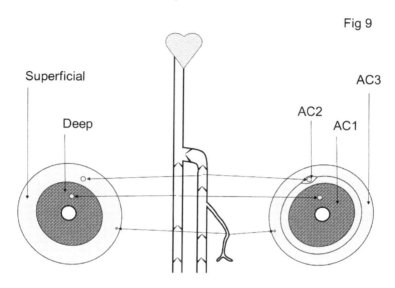

Fig 9

Figure 9: Diagram showing the different compartments of the leg, relevant to veins. On the left is what most doctors and nurses are taught – that there is only a deep and superficial system. On the right is the haemodynamically important orientation. The deep veins are in the muscle compartment – the deep or anatomical compartment 1 (AC1). The main truncal veins, called the saphenous veins, lie in the saphenous fascia, one of two superficial compartments called anatomical compartment 2 (AC2). Finally, the superficial veins lie in the second superficial compartment, anatomical compartment 3 (AC3). It is the fact that most doctors and nurses do not understand the difference between veins in the AC2 and those in the AC3 that there is so much confusion between different doctors and different treatments.

Therefore, we will consider the deep veins to be those veins that are buried deep inside the muscle. The superficial veins are the veins that lie between the skin and the muscle in the fat layer of the leg. Of course, the deep and superficial veins are linked. The two main superficial veins, the great saphenous vein and the small saphenous vein, both empty into the deep veins at well-defined junctions (Figure 10).

Fig 10

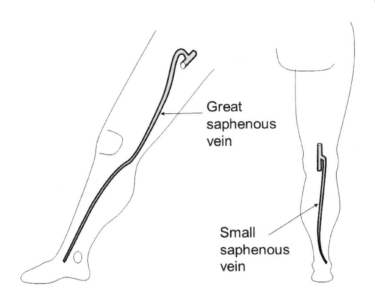

Figure 10: Diagram showing the 2 main truncal veins in the leg – the great and small saphenous veins. Before 2001, these were called the "long" and "short" saphenous veins. Anyone using these terms now is well over a decade out of date! It used to be thought that all venous disease that could be cured stemmed from these two veins. We now know that there are a great many other causes including the anterior accessory saphenous vein, incompetent perforating veins and pelvic veins, even before we start looking for less common causes. This huge number of possible sources of venous reflux is why detailed venous duplex ultrasound performed by a specially trained vascular technologist or clinical vascular scientist, is key to getting a correct diagnosis and hence proper treatment.

The great saphenous vein runs up the inner side of the leg, from ankle to groin, just under the skin. It finishes in the groin by diving deep into the leg and joins the deep vein at a junction. The deep vein is called the femoral vein at this point and so this junction is called the sapheno-femoral junction (SFJ).

The small saphenous vein runs up the back of the calf, and this vein finishes when it dives down deep into the leg behind the knee. At this point it joins the deep vein at a junction. The deep vein is called the popliteal vein at this point, and so the junction is called the sapheno-popliteal junction (SPJ).

Most doctors and nurses who treat varicose veins and leg ulcers only think about these two veins as "superficial veins" and then think about the deep veins separately. However, there are over 150 other communicating veins called perforators. They are called perforators because they "perforate" the muscle, running from the superficial veins into the deep veins. They only flow one way when the valves are working normally – from superficial to deep. Of course, when the valves stop working, these veins can also reflux. In this case, the venous reflux is not running down the vein by gravity but is squirting out of the deep veins into the superficial veins, because of muscle contraction. However, more about that later.

Venous leg pump

In order to pump blood upwards, from feet to heart, against gravity, two things are needed.

Firstly, there must be sufficient pressure pushing on the deep veins to force the blood upwards and out of the feet and lower legs, and towards the heart.

Secondly, there have to be one-way valves inside the veins to stop the blood from falling back down the veins once it has been pumped upwards.

To go through the first of these points, as discussed in the last chapter there are several pumps in the leg that push the blood up through the veins, towards the heart. These are all activated by movement. Standing up and putting weight on the foot, causes the foot to spread. The veins in the foot get stretched, squashing blood upwards into the calf. Contraction of the calf during walking or wiggling the ankle squashes the calf veins, pumping the blood up into the thigh and pelvis. Finally, contraction of the thigh muscles causes blood to be shot up into the pelvis (Figure 8).

Fig 11

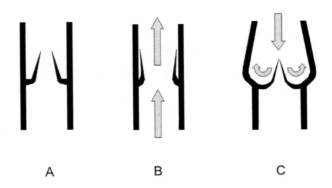

A   B   C

Figure 11: Diagram showing how a single venous valve works. A – at rest, there are 2 valve leaflets which look and act like little pockets pointing upwards. B – when venous blood is pumped upwards, the leaflets are forced apart by the venous blood flow. C – when the muscle pump relaxes, the blood falls back down the vein due to gravity. The reverse flow catches the valve leaflet, and as the blood collects in the "pocket" behind the valve leaflet, the valve snaps shut. This stops any further venous reflux. (Reproduced with consent from: "Understanding Venous Reflux: The Cause of Varicose Veins and Venous Leg Ulcers by Mark Whiteley)

Once the movement has completed, and the muscles relax, it would be a waste of time if the venous blood fell back down the veins to where it had started from. Therefore, all the veins in the legs have valves positioned some 8 to 10 cm apart. These valves are like pockets on a duffel coat. Each valve has two pockets with the open part facing upwards (Figure 11). When blood is forced through the valve, these valve leaflets or pockets are forced against the vein wall, letting the blood flow through. When the muscles relax and the blood tries to fall backwards down the leg by gravity, the blood gets caught in these pockets making the leaflets open, blocking the vein and stopping the blood falling downwards.

When the valves are working normally, the vein is said to be "competent".

Venous reflux

In a great many people, the valves in the veins fail (Figure 12). The exact causes are not known, but without doubt there is a hereditary component to this. We know this because studies show that things like varicose veins and venous leg ulcers tend to run in families.

One valve in one leg vein, failing by itself, is unlikely to cause a problem. However, if a series of valves in the same vein fail, then a column of blood can fall down the vein with gravity. When this happens, it is called venous reflux, as the blood is "refluxing" back down the vein rather than flowing up it. When a vein is allowing blood to reflux down it, the vein is called incompetent.

When venous reflux occurs in an incompetent vein, it means that when venous blood is pumped out of the leg, some of the venous blood falls back down the leg to where it started from. Consequently, the normal veins in the legs have to work even harder to push this blood back up towards the heart again, in addition to pumping all of the new blood coming into the leg from the arteries (Figure 13).

49

Fig 12

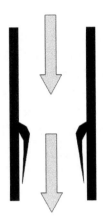

Figure 12: Diagram showing what happens when the venous valves "fail". The valve leaflets stop holding the refluxing blood and cannot shut anymore. This allows the blood to fall down the vein unimpeded ("venous reflux"). The valve, and this section of vein, are both said to be "incompetent". (Reproduced with consent from: "Understanding Venous Reflux: The Cause of Varicose Veins and Venous Leg Ulcers by Mark Whiteley)

More important than just making the other veins in the leg work harder, research has shown that as this blood falls down the veins, it hits the small veins around the ankles causing inflammation in the walls. This inflammation in the walls of the veins is the same sort of damage that is caused by stagnant blood in stasis veins. The body doesn't distinguish between inflammation caused by the impact of blood falling down the veins due to venous reflux, from inflammation due to stagnant blood getting more acidic and full of waste products. Both cause inflammation of the veins around the ankle and the surrounding tissues.

Of course, the body reacts to venous reflux to try and stop this inflammation and damage at the ankles. The way the body does this is to put "shock absorbers" into the incompetent vein

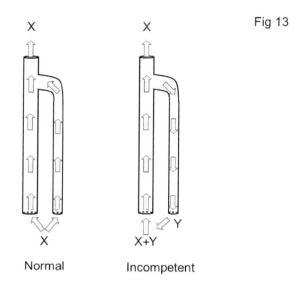

X   X   Fig 13

Y

X   X+Y

Normal   Incompetent

Figure 13: Diagram showing why venous reflux in an incompetent superficial vein causes swelling and overload of the veins at the foot and ankle. In the normal veins on the left, X amount of blood arriving in the foot from the arteries is pumped up both the deep and superficial veins, so that X amount is pumped out of the leg. However, in the incompetent system on the right, X amount of blood arriving in the veins in the foot from the arteries is pumped up the deep veins – but on relaxation, Y amount falls back down the incompetent superficial venous truncal vein. Now when the next X amount of blood arrives from the arteries, there is already Y amount of blood in the veins in the foot. Now the deep veins have to pump X and Y to get X out of the leg, as Y falls back down the veins again. Not only are the deep veins having to pump more than their fair share, but also there is always excessive amounts of venous blood in the foot when standing.

system. These shock absorbers try to stop the refluxing blood from hitting the ankle veins all at once, which is the cause of the inflammation. By allowing small veins that arise from the side of the large veins to dilate, some of the refluxing blood gets caught up in these dilated veins. As some of the refluxing blood gets way-laid in these dilated side-veins, the amount of blood hitting the ankle at one time reduces, and this reduces the inflammation caused at the ankle.

The balance of how much blood gets caught up in these dilated veins versus how much blood is allowed to reflux to cause inflammation at the ankles varies between different people. This is why different people with venous reflux present with different conditions. Those that have big bulging veins that are visible have "varicose veins" whereas those that get inflammation at the ankle get skin damage and venous leg ulcers. The underlying cause is the same for both (Figure 14).

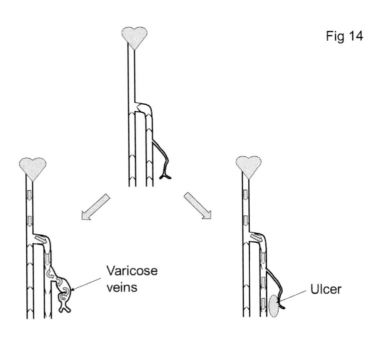

Fig 14

Varicose veins

Ulcer

Figure 14: Diagram answering the nonsensical question "Do varicose veins cause leg ulcers?" As shown here, reflux in the superficial truncal vein can either cause varicose veins, or a venous leg ulcer. Both are the results of superficial venous reflux. They may even co-exist. However, one does not cause the other.

What is really interesting is that in the past, people have thought that varicose veins are "just cosmetic", whereas venous leg ulcers are a serious medical condition! Even more interesting is that most people have thought that varicose veins are curable whereas venous leg ulcers are not! Hopefully, now you can see that both varicose veins and venous leg ulcers are usually caused by exactly the same underlying condition.

This has really blown the world of venous surgery apart as it means that:

1] varicose veins are not "just cosmetic" as they are a sign of underlying venous reflux which can go on to cause skin damage and leg ulceration
2] venous leg ulcers can be cured permanently by performing varicose vein type surgery

It is a major problem in medicine that doctors and nurses still make diagnoses by what they see. If they see bulging veins, they diagnose varicose veins. If they see a leg ulcer and no bulging veins, they diagnose a leg ulcer, without thinking that there may be a curable underlying vein condition. As nowadays venous reflux can be cured simply under local anaesthetic, curing most leg ulcers has become quite an easy thing for venous specialists to do.

In order to help health professionals to understand this, I introduced the term "hidden varicose veins" in about 2009. "Hidden varicose veins" is venous reflux in superficial veins that do not show any varicose veins on the surface. Medically it is often called superficial venous reflux (SVR), superficial venous incompetence (SVI) or chronic venous incompetence (CVI). However, "hidden varicose veins" is much easier and instantly tells people what it is. This phrase is slowly catching on and I would suggest that everyone use it for these patients, to keep reminding us that they are curable.

Finally, patients who do have venous reflux and venous leg ulcers always have dilated veins. As we have said, if these are visible on the surface these are called varicose veins. However, when they lie deep under the surface and often under the ulcer itself, these dilated veins allow venous blood to stagnate within them. This is the source of venous stasis in patients with venous reflux, whether they have "varicose veins" or "hidden varicose veins".

Deep versus superficial venous reflux

Before the mid-1980s, it was widely thought that patients with leg ulcers had reflux in their deep veins, and patients with varicose veins had reflux in the superficial veins. As it was impossible to treat deep veins then, it meant that people with venous leg ulcers could only be treated by compression. It also meant that people with varicose veins only had cosmetic problems, and they could have these treated if they wanted to, but it was not essential (Figure 15).

However, research in the mid-1980s and early 1990's showed that this was completely wrong.

The reason that everything changed was that in the mid-1980s, a new technique to investigate patients was invented. This was called venous duplex ultrasound.

Venous duplex ultrasound

It is beyond this simple book to go into detail about venous duplex ultrasound. However, very simply, venous duplex ultrasound is able to do three things at once. Firstly, it uses a black-and-white ultrasound to show the veins, arteries, fat and muscle et cetera in the leg. This is very much like the ultrasound used to see a gallbladder or a baby.

The second thing that venous duplex ultrasound can do is that when a vein is seen, the computer in the venous duplex

Fig 15

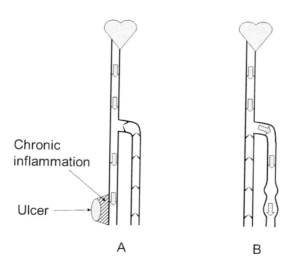

Chronic inflammation

Ulcer

A   B

Figure 15: Pre-1990, it used to be thought that deep vein reflux caused leg ulcers (A) and superficial venous reflux caused varicose veins (B). Despite many doctors and nurses still behaving as if this is the case, this was shown to be WRONG in the majority of cases in the 1990's.

ultrasound machine can tell whether there is any blood flow within it. More importantly, it can tell which way any blood is flowing and how fast. By using some very clever computing techniques, the venous duplex ultrasound machine represents this flow by putting red or blue colour onto the screen.

When an expert vascular technologist performs a venous duplex ultrasound, they can pressurise the venous blood by squeezing the calf and can watch the blood flow up the leg in a normal manner. If the patient is standing or sitting, releasing the pressure by letting go of the calf will allow the blood to start to fall down the vein. This of course will cause the valves to close and so no flow will be seen. The vein is said to be competent.

However, if the valves have failed, then blood will reflux down the vein, and this will be seen by colour flow on the screen, shown within the vein. The colour will be the opposite of the colour selected for the upward normal flow. In other words, if the computer was set to show blue flow upwards when the calf was squeezed, then if blood refluxed down the vein because the valves weren't working, it would appear red once the squeeze on the calf was relaxed.

Provided the patient is in a sitting or standing position, this venous reflux can be seen relatively easily by an experienced technologist. The deep veins and the superficial veins can all be examined. Therefore, venous reflux can be identified in deep and/or superficial veins, and reports can be made as to which veins are competent and which are incompetent.

The third component of the venous duplex ultrasound scan is the ability to measure the speed of flow using Doppler. However, this is only used rarely in vein surgery and we do not need to discuss this further in this book.

It is important to state at this point, although we will discuss this in more detail later, that we can also see perforator veins and flow within them. Flow in perforator veins should always be going from superficial to deep. However, sometimes even these valves can fail and blood can flow outwards under high pressure during muscle contraction, causing a different sort of venous reflux from the reflux down the superficial veins by gravity.

As reflux down the main veins requires gravity, venous duplex scanning does not show reflux if the patient is lying flat. Therefore, you cannot make a diagnosis of a competent or incompetent vein if the patient is lying flat. In venous surgery, we only look for clots when the patient is lying flat. Identification of venous reflux requires the patient to be sitting or standing.

It is very interesting that over the years, I have seen many patients who have been given the wrong advice and sometimes even the wrong treatment by doctors elsewhere, who perform their own venous duplex ultrasonography. In some cases, they perform this test with the patient lying flat. It is important for patients to know that the guidelines state that doctors should work in teams, and that in these teams, venous duplex ultrasonography must be available. Also all of the different techniques to treat the veins must be available (NICE CG 168 – July 2013). A doctor working by themselves and doing their own duplex scan is not following these guidelines and patients should be careful about any diagnosis or advice given.

Deep versus superficial venous reflux - continued

In the mid-1980s, when doctors who treat leg ulcers and varicose veins got their hands on duplex ultrasound, they started to investigate their patients' veins.

As with all new tests, doctors started using it to prove what they already thought that they knew. They expected the new venous duplex scans to show that their patients with venous leg ulcers would all have deep vein reflux, and their patients with varicose veins would all have superficial vein reflux.

Therefore, it came as a great surprise when the first couple of research papers were published showing that patients with venous leg ulcers often had the same pattern of venous reflux as patients with varicose veins. In other words, the previously held conviction that a venous leg ulcer was always caused by deep vein problems was wrong in many cases.

This research led us to the conclusions we have stated above - that varicose veins are not "just cosmetic" and venous leg ulcers are often curable by varicose vein type surgery.

Perforators and active/passive reflux

There is one last thing we have to think about when we talk about venous reflux. This is something that most doctors and nurses still do not understand. I have written several research papers to try and help them comprehend the role of perforators in venous disease, in order that they will start looking for these veins and start treating those that need treatment, so that their patients will get better results.

It is quite easy to imagine that when you stand up, blood can fall down a vein by gravity if there are no working valves to stop it. This is called passive reflux in my previous book on venous reflux, although many doctors and scientists in the world insist on calling this "diastolic" reflux. I personally do not like this term as I think of diastole as the relaxation of the heart, rather than the filling of veins on standing up.

However, this sort of reflux only happens in the great saphenous vein and a smaller associated vein called the anterior accessory vein in the leg, and the pelvic veins in the abdomen and pelvis

Fig 16

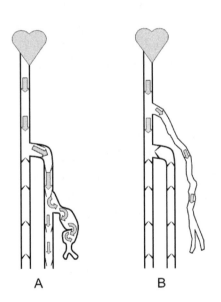

A   B

Figure 16: Passive reflux (also called "diastolic" reflux) occurs in the great saphenous vein (A) and the pelvic veins (B). (Reproduced with consent from: "Understanding Venous Reflux: The Cause of Varicose Veins and Venous Leg Ulcers by Mark Whiteley)

(Figure 16). The reason is that there are no valves in any veins above the upper ends of these veins. Hence, when any of these veins lose their working valves, blood can reflux all of the way from the heart, straight down these veins and into the veins and tissues below them, causing dilation (varicose veins) and inflammation.

Fig 17

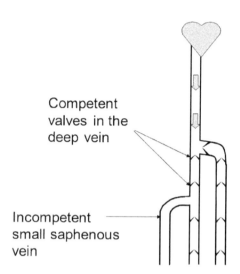

Competent
valves in the
deep vein

Incompetent
small saphenous
vein

Figure 17: Blood cannot reflux passively down an incompetent small saphenous vein from the heart on standing, if the valves are competent in the deep vein. They usually are competent! (Reproduced with consent from: "Understanding Venous Reflux: The Cause of Varicose Veins and Venous Leg Ulcers by Mark Whiteley)

This is different from the situation in the case of the small saphenous vein. As described above, the small saphenous vein runs up the back of the calf and joins with the deep veins behind the knee. Above this point, the deep vein in the thigh still contains valves, preventing a column of blood falling all the way from the heart to the ankle. In an incompetent small saphenous vein, a column of refluxing blood can only start from just behind the knee. As such, reflux in the small saphenous vein should not cause a problem (Figure 17).

However, every doctor who treats varicose veins knows that reflux in the small saphenous vein can cause bad varicose veins and treating the small saphenous vein can cure them. Therefore, this means that the venous reflux in the small saphenous vein is different than the simple passive reflux in the great saphenous vein.

The reason is that in the small saphenous vein, the venous reflux happens when the muscles are contracting, not when they are relaxed (Figure 18). As we discussed when talking about the

Fig 18

Incompetent
small
saphenous
reflux

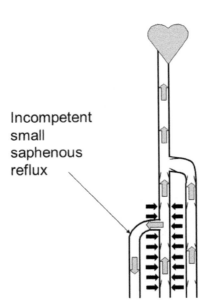

Figure 18: Blood refluxes down an incompetent small saphenous vein when muscles in the leg contract. Hence this is active reflux (also called "systolic" reflux). (Reproduced with consent from: "Understanding Venous Reflux: The Cause of Varicose Veins and Venous Leg Ulcers by Mark Whiteley)

vein pump, venous blood gets pumped out of the leg when the calf muscle contracts. This forces blood under high pressure up the deep veins to the heart.

However, if the valves have failed in the small saphenous vein, it will allow blood to be shot out of the deep veins and down this superficial vein under high pressure, during muscle contraction. The effect of this high-pressure wave is the same as a volume of blood refluxing by passive reflux down the great saphenous vein from the heart. The energy of the blood being forced down this vein will impact in the small veins and tissues at the bottom of the vein, causing inflammation.

The body will react by dilating side veins to try and stop this. Once again this will result in either varicose veins, or the inflammation of the tissues resulting in red stains, brown stains, hardness or leg ulcers. Therefore, the end result of the venous reflux is the same, although the mechanism of the reflux is different.

Because this reflux depends upon muscle contraction, I have called this "active" reflux in my previous book, although once again, other workers in the field call this "systolic" reflux. My objections to this term are the same as above.

If you can imagine how active reflux works in the small saphenous vein, and can see the consequences of it, then you will be able to understand what happens if a valve fails in a perforator vein (Figure 19).

Reflux in a perforator vein only occurs when the muscles contract. As most tests for venous reflux look for reflux after compression of the muscle (i.e. in the relaxation phase), then most current tests miss perforator vein reflux. This is probably why it has not been understood in the past and why most doctors and nurses still do not understand it.

Fig 19

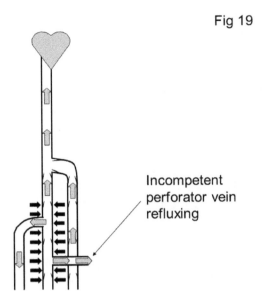

Incompetent
perforator vein
refluxing

Figure 19: Incompetent perforating veins also reflux actively ("systolic" reflux). However, despite most surgeons knowing that an incompetent small saphenous vein can cause varicose veins, skin damage or even leg ulcers, most still do not look for, nor treat, incompetent perforating veins!

Another reason that perforator vein reflux has largely been ignored in the medical world is that these small veins are difficult to treat. Doctors tend to ignore things they do not want to treat. However, in 2001, Judy Holdstock and I invented the transluminal occlusion of perforator (TRLOP) technique. Using TRLOP, we can close these incompetent perforator veins under local anaesthetic using ultrasound to guide us and only using a single needle hole. This has been "reinvented" in the United States as the "perforator ablation procedure" (PAPS) by a doctor who saw me present TRLOP in the early 2000's. PAPS is exactly the same as TRLOP. It was given a different name by the person "describing" it, several years after we had already published our long-term results.

Increasing amounts of research has now shown that closing the incompetent perforators increases the chance of curing venous leg ulcers. Hence, it is essential for anyone working in the field of venous leg ulcers to be able to identify incompetent perforators with venous duplex ultrasonography and to be able to perform the TRLOP technique to ablate them.

However, we will come back to treatment in a later chapter.

In this chapter, we have had a whistle-stop tour of venous reflux. We have discussed deep and superficial venous reflux as well as active and passive reflux. We have shown how venous reflux causes inflammation or varicose veins. We have looked at the difference in reflux in the great saphenous vein from that in the small saphenous vein. We have shown that both small saphenous vein reflux and perforator vein reflux can also be associated with venous leg ulcers.

We are now going to have a brief look at the less common problem of venous obstruction before we move on to look at how we can treat the veins and cure venous leg ulcers permanently.

Chapter 5

Venous obstruction

It is very easy to get confused between veins and arteries. You often hear people talking about "blocked veins" when they are discussing varicose veins. Hopefully, if you have followed the words and diagrams in chapter 4, you will now understand that most venous problems are due to reflux. This is the failure of valves and nothing to do with any narrowing or blockages in the veins.

We are now going to discuss venous obstruction which, fortunately, is very uncommon in patients with venous leg ulcers. However, now that it is often curable, it is essential that we talk about it in this book.

What is venous obstruction?

Simply, venous obstruction is a narrowing or complete blockage of the vein. If blocked, the blood has to find another route back to the heart. If narrowed, the resistance to flow is so great that once again blood has to find another route back to the heart.

Of course, as we have pointed out previously, because of gravity blood does not flow out of the leg naturally, unless the person is lying down. It has to be pumped by the muscle pumps in the leg, and once pumped up the veins, valves have to keep the venous blood at the level that it has been pumped to.

If there is a venous obstruction in one of the major veins of the legs or pelvis, then blood cannot get out of the leg by the normal route when being pumped during walking (Figure 20).

Fig 20

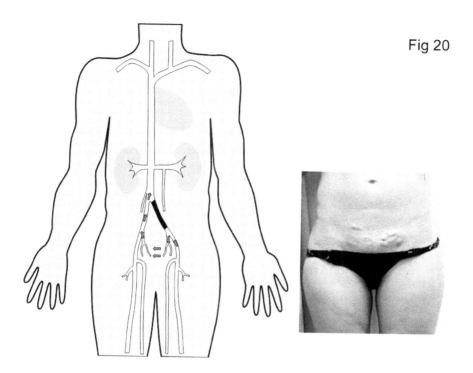

Figure 20: The very uncommon condition of a blocked pelvic vein can cause varicose veins. But such varicose veins are usually in abnormal places such as across the pubic area (as shown) or up the flanks.

This can lead to several problems.

Clearly if the blood is not getting out of the leg easily, the leg usually swells. For the same reason, the veins often dilate showing varicose veins on the surface or "hidden varicose veins" under the surface. This includes the veins low down around the ankle where blood can stagnate causing "stasis veins". As we have seen, stasis veins can result in inflammation around the ankle with the usual red stains, brown stains, hardness of the skin around the ankles or even venous leg ulcers.

As the blood cannot be forced easily out of the leg during walking, this ends up with a back pressure when the muscles are

65

pumping, causing the patient to get a cramping pain and to stop walking. This is called "venous claudication".

What causes venous obstruction?

The commonest cause of venous obstruction is a previous thrombosis in the vein (DVT) that has resulted in the vein wall being damaged, scarred and either narrowed or blocked.

Research presented by Prof Vaughan Ruckley in Edinburgh two decades ago showed that if you have only had one DVT in the past, and this has been treated quickly, then it rarely causes a problem in your deep veins. However, the more DVTs you have, and the longer they take to be resolved, the more scar tissue is likely to accumulate.

Many doctors and nurses still think that if you have a DVT, it causes the valves to fail in the deep veins causing deep vein reflux. However, research from the United States from Dr Raju and Dr Nieglen have shown that even when a venous duplex ultrasound scan suggests that there is deep vein reflux causing a leg ulcer, careful examination shows that this is usually secondary to a venous obstruction higher up in the venous system.

You might wonder why this is important.

The reason that this has become important is that a venous obstruction in the pelvic veins can now be treated with a high chance of success, by putting a balloon through the blockage and placing a stent into the vein. This can open a blocked vein or a narrowed vein, keeping it permanently open. Patients in my own practice who have had this done have ended up with legs going from being excessively swollen to being normal or almost normal size, venous leg ulcers disappearing, patients restricted to short distances of walking being able to get back to long walks or even running.

It is suggested that 90% of people with "deep vein reflux"

actually have venous obstruction and a large proportion of these might be treatable with stents. It must be said that this is an active area of research and results are improving all of the time.

Fig 21

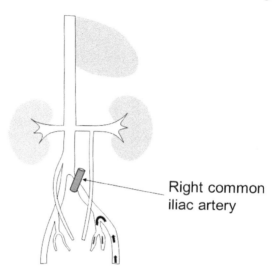

Right common
iliac artery

Figure 21: This diagram shows a classic May-Thurner syndrome. The right common iliac artery crosses over the left common iliac vein, crushing it against the spine and causing an obstruction. This used to be thought to be a common condition. However, we are now finding that although some tests show a narrowing here, it rarely causes a real problem.

Conversely, in the 10% who have deep vein reflux without obstruction, there is still no way to form an artificial valve. These patients, along with the ones that have obstruction that cannot be stented, are now amongst the only patients with venous leg ulceration that cannot be cured with modern techniques.

There are other causes of venous obstruction and the most commonly known one in the medical world is the May-Thurner syndrome (Figure 21). This occurs when the vein in the pelvis on the left side gets squashed by an artery crossing over the front of it, trapping it against the spine. In fact, this does not occur anywhere near as commonly as previously thought. There are also other conditions called non-thrombotic iliac vein lesions (NIVL) that can also cause narrowing and DVT on either side. However, whatever the cause of any narrowing or blockages, the investigations and treatments are the same.

Chapter 6

Investigations for venous leg ulcers

When investigating a patient with a venous leg ulcer, there are two general areas to think about:

1] the general health of the patient
2] the investigations of what is the underlying cause
   of the leg ulcer

General health of the patient

Most doctors, nurses and healthcare professionals are very good at assessing the general health of the patient.

As far as venous leg ulcers are concerned, the most important thing to assess is the ability to move the ankle and secondary to that, the ability to walk.

If you have been reading this book in order, you will by now have realised the importance of the venous leg pump. This has two components, the movement and the valves.

In the next few chapters we are going to talk about the treatments of the veins by correcting the problems caused by valve failure. However, there is no point in even considering any such treatment if there is no movement to start the venous pumping again.

Therefore, patients who are bedbound or who are not going to get back to walking again are not going to be put forward for any of the venous surgical techniques that we are going to discuss in the next couple of chapters, with perhaps the only exception of foam sclerotherapy for any stasis veins.

Bedbound patients should be treated with elevation and, if sitting out of bed, with either external compression of the leg or an external pump, to give the veins some element of venous pump function.

However, patients who are able to walk should be fully and actively investigated, provided they have no other serious or terminal disease that would prevent them from undergoing treatment under local anaesthetic. Any low-protein states or other curable disease should be treated as soon as possible in order to get the best possible result from treatment to cure the leg ulcer.

In view of the protein loss from the weeping of a leg ulcer, and the use of vitamin C by the body when it is trying to heal, I always advise my patients to start vitamin C 1000 mg a day whilst they have their leg ulcer and to continue it every day until the ulcer is cured. I also advise a high-protein diet so that they have the building blocks to build new cells and tissue during the healing process.

Investigation of the underlying cause of a leg ulcer

It is sad that most doctors, nurses and healthcare professionals treating people with leg ulcers, although good at assessing the general health and mobility of patients, are very bad at assessing the cause of the leg ulcer itself.

Most perform a "Doppler test". This is merely a blood pressure cuff placed around the calf, and then a hand held Doppler machine is used to listen to blood flow in the arteries around the ankle or foot. The blood pressure cuff is pumped up and when the flow of blood is heard, the doctor, nurse or health care professional is able to measure the pressure of blood in the arteries.

The only use for this Doppler test is to see if there is any arterial insufficiency. As we have already seen, this only occurs in 10% of leg ulcers. We can also get the same information by looking at the position of the leg ulcers on the lower leg, asking the patient if they get pain in the leg or foot at night, and by observing the changes in the foot when lifting the leg up when the patient is lying down. If there is good arterial pressure, the toes will still be pink when the leg is raised. If the arterial pressure is poor, the toes go a deathly white when the leg is raised.

As most patients with leg ulcers have venous leg ulcers, we now have to think about the investigations for patients with venous leg ulcers.

Venous duplex ultrasound scanning

We have already talked about venous duplex ultrasound scanning in chapter 4. Simply, a black-and-white ultrasound image can be seen on the ultrasound machine, showing the vein as well as any surrounding structures such as arteries, fat, muscle and skin.

Using the Doppler technology within the machine, the ultrasound machine can then detect flow, superimposing a red or blue colour onto the vein to show which way the blood is flowing.

If there is a clot such as a DVT, there will be no flow. If the patient is laid flat and the vein is pushed with the ultrasound probe, a normal vein will squash flat. However, a vein that is full of clot will not squash flat. The combination of no flow in a vein and the fact it cannot be squashed means there is a clot within the vein. If this is a deep vein, it is a DVT. If it is a superficial vein, it is a superficial venous thrombosis that is usually called "phlebitis".

If the patient is sitting upright or standing, then there is now gravity affecting the blood in the veins.

Using the free hand to squeeze the calf muscle, it is possible to use the duplex ultrasound machine to see blood flowing up the veins. When the pressure on the calf muscle is released, blood starts to flow back down the veins due to gravity. If the valves are working, the valves close and the blood does not fall down the veins. This shows a competent vein. However, if the valves have failed, the blood can reflux down the vein. The duplex ultrasound scan shows this reversed flow as the opposite colour within the vein. This vein is then diagnosed as incompetent.

When we are investigating the small saphenous vein and incompetent perforating veins, we have to check the reflux during compression as well, as reflux can occur during the compression phase (active reflux). However, as pushing on the muscle is not the same as muscle contraction, both the compression and the relaxation phase are checked. Provided the blood always flows in the direction that it should (either up the vein or inwards from superficial to deep) then there is no reflux. Reflux is diagnosed when blood flows the wrong way through the vein.

By using these techniques, vascular technologists and vascular scientists are able to get very accurate diagnoses as to the state of the deep and superficial veins in the legs. It is possible to diagnose deep vein obstruction or reflux, superficial vein reflux and perforator vein reflux. We can also find stasis veins under the damaged skin or venous leg ulcer.

Research presented in New York in 2014 showed that if a doctor does their own scan, and they do other things such as surgery and consult patients, then they can miss up to 30% of the venous problems. This is because they do not specialise in the scan techniques and do not perform venous duplex examinations all day, every day. As such, recommendations are that venous doctors should work in teams and not try to be an individual who does the diagnosis and treatment all by themselves.

In the great majority of cases, the diagnosis from the venous duplex ultrasound scan performed by a specially trained vascular technologist or clinical vascular scientist who specialises in the venous system, will be sufficient to be able to tell us whether the patient is curable, and more importantly, what technique or series of techniques are needed to cure the patient.

Air plethysmography

Uncommonly, the duplex may suggest that the deep veins are refluxing or that there is more disease than the duplex appears to show. In these patients, we may consider that there might be venous obstruction. We often call this "outflow obstruction" or "venous outflow obstruction".

If the venous obstruction is in the deep veins in the leg, this will be shown by venous duplex ultrasound. Therefore, it is really only venous obstruction in the pelvic veins that cannot be seen easily by venous duplex ultrasound scanning.

In these patients it is always tempting to do magnetic resonance imaging (MRI) which is often called magnetic resonance venography (MRV), or CT scanning, or venography. There is even a very sophisticated ultrasound that is performed from inside the vein using a tiny probe on the end of a catheter called "intravascular ultrasound" (IVUS). The problem with all of these techniques is that they tend to show the anatomy rather than the function. They are very useful if we know there is a functional problem and we are merely looking for where the problem is.

Air plethysmography is a technique where a blood pressure cuff is placed around the lower leg and inflated to quite a low pressure. This is attached to a machine that measures the volume of air inside the cuff.

The patient starts off standing up. They are then either tipped upside down or, more commonly, lie on their back and lift their leg up in the air. In a normal person, the blood will fall by gravity straight out of the leg, through the veins of the pelvis and back to the right heart. This will result in the calf shrinking quickly and the machine showing a very fast decrease in calf volume ("waterfall emptying") (Figure 22).

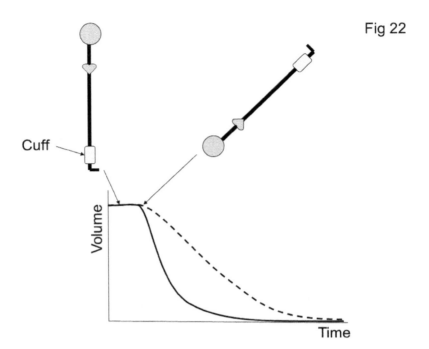

Figure 22: Diagram showing how air-plethysmography is used to test for venous obstruction. A cuff is inflated around the calf to monitor the volume of the lower leg. The patient starts standing. The volume reaches a stable value. The patient is then tipped upside down (or lies down quickly, lifting the leg in the air). A normal vein will allow the leg to empty quickly (solid line). An obstructed vein will hold up the flow, slowing down the rate of venous emptying (dotted line).

If there is any venous obstruction, the blood will not be able to fall out of the leg so easily when performing the same manoeuvre. The blood will have to flow through smaller veins, bypassing the problem, to try to get back to the heart. This slow emptying results in the calf decreasing in volume at a much slower rate. This is measured by the machine showing a slow calf emptying curve.

This simple and relatively inexpensive test gives a very good idea of whether there is significant venous obstruction or not.

74

Of course, it can also be used in reverse. Once the patient is lying on their back with their leg up, they can then stand up. If all of the valves in the legs are working, then the leg has to fill through arterial blood supply. The blood has to go from the arteries through the capillaries and slowly fill the veins. This will mean that the cuff shows a very slow filling of the leg.

However, if the valves in the veins are not working (superficial or deep) then venous blood will fall rapidly back down the leg by reflux and the cuff will show that the leg has expanded rapidly.

In this way, air plethysmography can be used to look both for venous obstruction as well as venous reflux of the legs.

Uncommonly, we do still use other investigations such as MRV, CT, venography or IVUS, but really these are rarely needed these days. We only need these when we are trying to identify the position of an obstruction that has been shown on air plethysmography.

Now we are going to move on to discuss how we can cure venous leg ulcers.

Chapter 7

Principles of treatment

As we have seen in previous chapters, the reason that patients get venous leg ulcers is because of inflammation. This inflammation is in the veins and surrounding tissues, low down in the leg, by the ankle.

Not surprisingly, all treatments for venous leg ulcers aim to reduce this inflammation. Whether it is the temporary healing of dressing and bandaging or the permanent cure of local anaesthetic surgery techniques, everything that works only works because it reduces this inflammation.

Therefore, before going on to consider different treatments in more detail, it is worth thinking about inflammation a bit more.

Inflammation

Most people have a fairly good idea of what is meant by "inflammation". When we hurt ourselves by falling over or trapping a finger in a door, or develop a boil or local infection, we get a hot, red, swollen area that is painful. When we have such an area on our body, we know instantly that this is "inflamed".

Unfortunately though, when most people see an area that is red, hot, swollen and painful, they instantly think it is an infection. Even worse, most doctors and nurses jump to the same conclusion.

Of course, this is not always correct.

If you were punched on the nose, your nose would go red, hot, swollen and painful. The fact you knew you had been punched would stop you from assuming that it was an infection of the nose. However, the nose is still inflamed but because you know what caused it, you don't jump to the conclusion it is infected.

This tells us a lot about inflammation.

The body reacts to anything that damages it by inflammation. There are many different ways that the body can be damaged. It can be damaged by physical trauma, infection, chemical burns, thermal burns - even some cancers. You will note that only one of these causes is infection.

In all cases, the reaction that is seen from the inflammation is the same:

- Redness
- Heat
- Swelling
- Pain

The reason that the body responds to any such damage with inflammation is because inflammation is how the body protects itself and then heals.

When something starts to damage cells or tissues in the body, the local tissues react by releasing some special chemicals. These chemicals are called "inflammatory mediators".

These inflammatory mediators, released from the tissues around the area of damage, affect the local blood vessels. They cause the local arterial blood vessels to dilate, bringing more blood into the local area. Because more arterial blood flows into the area, this naturally brings more white blood cells into the vicinity of the problem.

White blood cells fight infection and remove damaged tissues. They do this by a combination of making antibodies, killing and "eating" infective germs, or removing bad cells or damaged tissue.

A side effect of increasing the local arterial blood flow is that the area goes red and gets hotter. This is because arterial blood comes straight from the heart at high pressure and is hotter than the limbs and surface of the body.

The next action of the inflammatory mediators is that they make the local capillaries become "leaky". Capillaries are the tiny blood vessels that lie in networks through all tissues and organs in the body. It is through the capillaries that oxygen and nutrients can pass from the blood into the tissues, and carbon dioxide and waste products diffuse back into the blood.

When the capillaries become leaky, the fluid part of blood which is called plasma can leak through the capillary walls, leaving the blood and going outside of the blood vessels and into the local tissues. If this occurs at the surface of the body, such as in a graze or in an ulcer, this fluid leaks out onto the surface. As we saw previously, the aim is for the water to evaporate leaving the protein to form a scab. In other cases, when the skin is intact, or the inflammation is deeper in the body, the fluid collects locally around the area of the tissue damage. This increase in the local liquid causes the swelling of inflammation.

This fluid release is a very important part of the inflammatory process. As noted above, if this fluid is released from a break in the surface, it can form a scab allowing the surface to heal. When the fluid collects deeper in the body, it dilutes any toxins or damaging chemicals. It also acts as a space for the white cells to move out of the blood vessels and get to work on invading microbes or damaged tissue.

Finally, some of the inflammatory mediators cause pain in the local tissues. This is essential as it is pain that stops patients from moving or touching the affected area, allowing the body to get on with the job of healing.

Hence it is a shame that when most doctors, nurses or healthcare professionals see inflammation, they almost always think there is an infection. The result is that they often take a swab and prescribe antibiotics! In many cases, this is not the right thing to do as the inflammation is often due to non-infective causes.

Chronic inflammation

Although inflammation is the way the body reacts to reduce damage and heal itself, this all changes if the process of inflammation cannot remove the damage that is causing it in the first place. In other words, if you have been punched and the trauma is over, then inflammation will heal the damaged tissues. The same can be said for healing from a graze or having a surgical operation. The inflammation allows the body to heal because the thing that caused the inflammation in the first place has stopped and been removed.

This is also true for infections. If the inflammation successfully removes the invading microorganism, sometimes by killing it and ingesting it, other times by forming pus which is expelled from the body, then the inflammation can let the tissues heal themselves.

However, if something starts inflammation off in some tissues, and the inflammation cannot get rid of the underlying cause, then more inflammation is caused on top of the inflammatory process that has already started. In this case, the inflammation continues in the long term. When this happens, it is called "chronic inflammation". Unlike inflammation that happens quickly and causes healing, this chronic inflammation can be very destructive.

Examples of the destruction that can be caused by chronic inflammation are conditions such as rheumatoid arthritis. In rheumatoid arthritis, chronic inflammation affects the joints and often ends up completely destroying the affected joints. The way to cure this would be to remove the cause of the inflammation. But in rheumatoid arthritis we can't do this.

This is because we don't actually know the precise cause of the inflammation. As we cannot remove the cause of the inflammation, we are left with only one option. We have to leave the chronic inflammation process alone, and try to damp down the inflammatory response, using anti-inflammatory drugs.

The principle is very similar to that in venous leg ulcers. Venous leg ulcers are caused by chronic inflammation of the tissues in the lower legs. As we have seen before, this chronic inflammation comes from the veins underlying the tissue being inflamed. We have already seen what the causes of this inflammation are. It can be the stagnant blood in the stasis veins underlying the ulcer. In addition to this, venous reflux, either passively falling down the long veins, or actively being pumped out through incompetent small saphenous veins or perforators, causes inflammation by the impact of the blood hitting the vein wall. Lastly, obstruction of the veins can increase stagnation and stasis.

Luckily for patients with venous leg ulcers, we can now identify reflux, stasis and obstruction in the veins using venous duplex ultrasound. Even more importantly, we can now usually cure the problem with techniques we will explain in the next chapters.

By removing the cause of the chronic inflammation, we stop any more inflammation being stimulated. The current inflammation can do its proper job of helping the body heal, letting the tissues go back to being normal and allowing the skin to grow back again. Once this healing process is completed, the inflammatory process completely stops as there is nothing causing any further chronic inflammation. The result of this is that the venous leg ulcers not only heal but are permanently cured.

This principle really is quite simple, and case after case that I've treated has shown this to be true. Indeed, we have even published our 12-years results from The Whiteley Clinic showing that we can completely cure 85% of venous ulcers using these principles.

Unfortunately, most patients don't get this opportunity. They end up being "treated" by having dressings put on the ulcer and then compression applied to the lower leg.

Dressings and compression appear to work in some patients in the short term. Compression on the veins of the lower leg will empty some of the stasis veins, reducing the amount of stagnant blood. By increasing the pressure using compression, the amount of venous reflux will reduce. Also, by increasing the pressure by compression, this extra venous pressure will help venous blood to leave the leg by forcing it through any obstruction. This is why people appear to heal their ulcers with compression therapy.

However, as soon as the compression is taken off, the stasis veins reopen increasing the amount of stagnant blood again, the venous reflux starts all over again and the obstruction is still there. Hence compression has done nothing but provide some temporary relief or temporary healing. It is never a cure in a venous leg ulcer.

Curing venous leg ulcers by stopping chronic inflammation

One of the wonderful things about medical science, is that once principles can be established, treatments can be devised that not only really work, but also have good long-term results. Failure to follow medical science means that practitioners follow practices that are "traditional ".

It is not really surprising that if you use the same techniques that were used 100 years ago, the results won't be significantly improved.

Over 100 years ago, patients with venous leg ulcers were treated with dressings and compression. Medical science has shown us that most of these patients have their ulcers because of reflux, stasis and/or obstruction - and has also shown us how to cure these conditions.

Therefore, you would have thought it is blindingly obvious that to cure patients with venous leg ulcers, you need to correct these problems. It is amazing that the majority of professionals treating venous leg ulcers, still completely ignore this and continue dressings and compression as their standard approach.

As most of this medical science was worked out and published in the 1990s and early 2000's, we have known most of these principles for a couple of decades now. So, what is really surprising is that I have even had to write this book at all, and that I still have to give so many talks on this subject to professionals as if it were "new". You really would have thought that these proven techniques of investigating and treating the underlying veins that cause leg ulcers would have been adopted widely already.

So how do we cure venous leg ulcers?

In the most basic form:

- If there is reflux - stop the reflux
- If there are venous stasis veins - remove them so blood cannot stagnate
- If there is obstruction - get rid of the obstruction

Turning to the first of these, we need to stop venous reflux. As venous reflux is due to valves failing, the obvious way to treat this is to repair the valves or to replace them. Unfortunately, that is impossible. No-one has ever been able to repair venous valves successfully or make a reliable replacement valve for the leg veins.

Therefore, if it is impossible to repair the valves, the only way to stop venous reflux is to block the incompetent vein and stop any blood flowing through it. This would clearly stop the vein from refluxing. However, most patients that have come to see me, and most doctors and nurses that I teach, ask one question - "if you block the vein, where does the blood go?"

82

They get very concerned that permanently blocking a vein might have some detrimental effect on the body.

If you have followed this book so far, you will already know this is a ridiculous question. However, you wouldn't believe how many doctors or nurses try to explain this by saying "the blood finds another way". Anyone who says this does not understand veins and no patients should be treated by anyone who gives this as a serious answer to their question.

The answer is best explained using a model that I started telling patients in about 2004. In this model, we think about veins as a person using a bucket to lift water. I will explain this fully in the next chapter.

Chapter 8

Where does the blood go?

Curing venous leg ulcers permanently, treating varicose veins successfully and curing a great many other venous conditions depends upon stopping venous reflux effectively and permanently.

As explained at the end of the last chapter, we cannot make incompetent veins competent again, as we cannot repair the valves in a vein. Therefore, the only way we can stop venous reflux in a vein is to remove the vein or to block it off permanently.

Fig 23

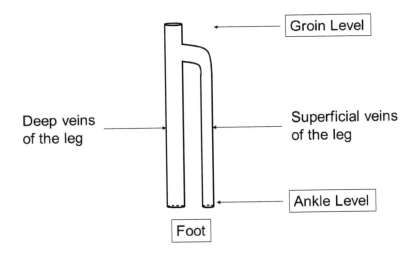

Figure 23: Explanation of "Where does the blood go if you remove or block off an incompetent vein". See text for details.

Fig 24

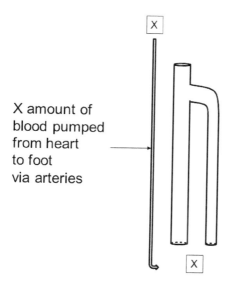

X amount of blood pumped from heart to foot via arteries

Figure 24: Explanation of "Where does the blood go if you remove or block off an incompetent vein". See text for details.

When I explain this to patients, the commonest question I get asked is "where does the blood go?" A great many patients worry that if you permanently remove or block a vein, it may cause a problem.

Of course, this is not the case, provided the correct vein is treated. Over the many years that I have been asked this question, I have developed the following explanation to help patients, doctors and nurses understand the principles of venous reflux surgery.

Venous flow in deep and superficial veins

In the leg, thinking at the simplest level, we have deep veins running up inside the muscle and superficial veins running up under the skin (Figure 23). The superficial veins join with the deep veins in the groin (Figure 23).

However, you must remember that these are veins not arteries. It is the arteries that take blood to the foot whereas it is the job of these veins to bring blood back from the foot and take it back to the heart.

If we imagine that "X" amount of blood is pumped from the heart to the foot, we can think that there is X amount of blood that needs to be pumped back to the heart (Figure 24).

Therefore, X amount of blood needs to be pumped by the veins from the foot, out of the leg, into the pelvic veins and back to the heart (Figure 25). If less than X amount of blood is pumped out of the foot, then the foot would start to swell and go blue, as it filled up with blood. Therefore, if X amount of blood goes to

Fig 25

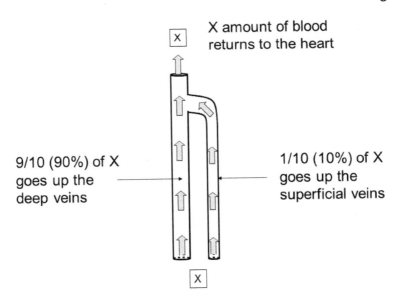

X amount of blood
returns to the heart

9/10 (90%) of X
goes up the
deep veins

1/10 (10%) of X
goes up the
superficial veins

Figure 25: Explanation of "Where does the blood go if you remove or block off an incompetent vein". See text for details.

86

the foot through the arteries, the veins in the leg have to expel X amount of blood from the leg, to keep the circulation in balance.

Research has shown us that the deep veins pump 9/10 (90%) of X. The superficial veins pump 1/10 (10%) of X (Figure 25).

So what people worry about is what happens if you remove or close the superficial veins (Figure 26). If you did this in a normal person, of course the deep veins would have to work harder

Fig 26

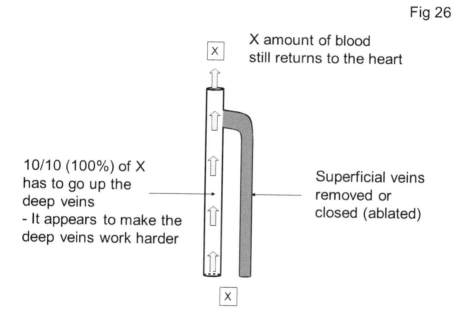

X amount of blood
still returns to the heart

10/10 (100%) of X
has to go up the
deep veins
- It appears to make the
deep veins work harder

Superficial veins
removed or
closed (ablated)

Figure 26: Explanation of "Where does the blood go if you remove or block off an incompetent vein". See text for details.

(Figure 26). However, you will be pleased to note this is not what actually happens. This is because we do not operate on people with normal veins!

Reflux in superficial veins

Thanks to venous duplex ultrasound scanning, we can now see which veins are incompetent. In patients with venous leg ulcers, the commonest cause is superficial venous incompetence. This is represented in Figure 27. You might be interested to know this is exactly the same situation as for people who have varicose veins.

As you can see in Figure 27, X amount of blood still has to be pumped out of the leg veins into the pelvis. Because the superficial vein is not competent, the deep vein has to pump the whole of X. However, the situation is even worse than that. As the superficial vein is incompetent, it is allowing a certain amount of blood that has already been pumped up the deep vein, to fall back down it into the foot.

If we think that the superficial veins allow Y amount of blood to reflux back down them, this means that the foot now has X

Fig 27

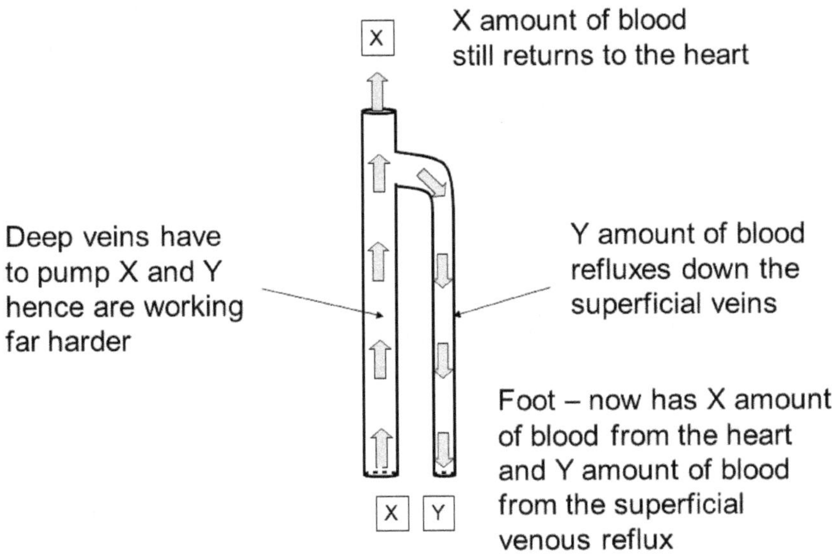

X amount of blood still returns to the heart

Deep veins have to pump X and Y hence are working far harder

Y amount of blood refluxes down the superficial veins

Foot – now has X amount of blood from the heart and Y amount of blood from the superficial venous reflux

Figure 27: Explanation of "Where does the blood go if you remove or block off an incompetent vein". See text for details.

Fig 28

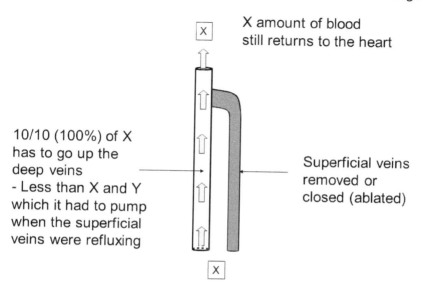

X amount of blood
still returns to the heart

10/10 (100%) of X
has to go up the
deep veins
- Less than X and Y
which it had to pump
when the superficial
veins were refluxing

Superficial veins
removed or
closed (ablated)

Figure 28: Explanation of "Where does the blood go if you remove or block off an incompetent vein". See text for details.

amount of blood arriving from the arteries, but also Y amount of blood falling back into the foot from the incompetent veins. Not surprisingly, as venous reflux gets worse over time, ankles start to swell (Figure 27).

In order to get X amount of blood out of the leg, the deep veins now have to pump the whole of X AND the whole of Y. In other words, the deep veins are having to overwork to compensate for the incompetent superficial veins.

Now we can see that when we remove or block off the superficial vein (Figure 28) this actually reduces the amount of blood that is in the foot, and it reduces the amount of work the deep vein has to do to get X amount of blood out of the foot. As we have seen above, this is not the case in normal veins, but is only the case when we are treating incompetent veins.

The bucket model

It is a very difficult concept to understand and I am sure that despite going through the above, some people will still have difficulty picturing this. I know that I did when I was developing my theories on venous disease.

When I was a junior doctor I never really understood venous reflux. Therefore, in the early 2000's, I developed the following model firstly for myself to understand what happens and secondly to try and explain venous reflux to patients. Fortunately, this model also answers the question "where does the blood go?"

Imagine the circulation system as a water tank filling a bath (Figure 29). The water tank above the bath represents the heart. This allows water to flow under pressure down the pipes, through the tap and into the bath. In this model, we can think of the bath as a leg, the pipes as arteries and the water as blood.

Fig 29

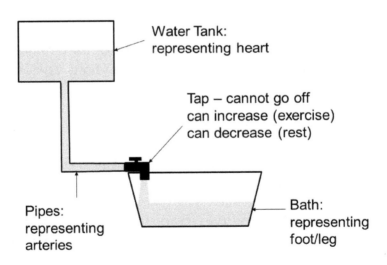

Figure 29: My "bucket" model to understand venous reflux. See text for details.

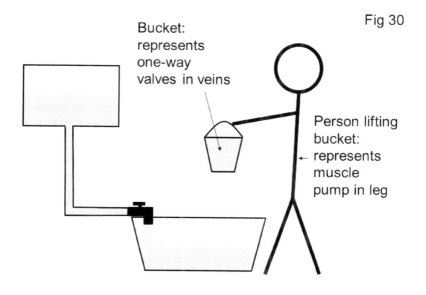

Fig 30

Bucket: represents one-way valves in veins

Person lifting bucket:
← represents muscle pump in leg

Figure 30: My "bucket" model to understand venous reflux. See text for details.

The tap is always on because we cannot stop blood flow to the leg. Of course, we can increase the flow when we exercise, and we can decrease it when we rest, but we cannot stop it completely.

This represents the arterial system feeding blood to the leg.

To represent the venous system, we have to return blood back to the tank from the bath. The easiest way to represent the veins in this model is to consider a person with a bucket, scooping water from the bath and putting it back into the tank (Figure 30). Although this is quite simplistic, it is amazing how accurately this represents the real situation.

The person provides the power to lift the water back to the tank. This is the same as the muscles in the leg pumping the blood back to the heart.

As we have discussed before, a pump only works if there are valves. In this model the bucket represents valves as it only allows the water to go one way i.e. upwards against gravity from bath to tank.

If you now imagine that for a certain flow of water through the tap, the person will have to work at a certain speed to keep the bath level maintained.

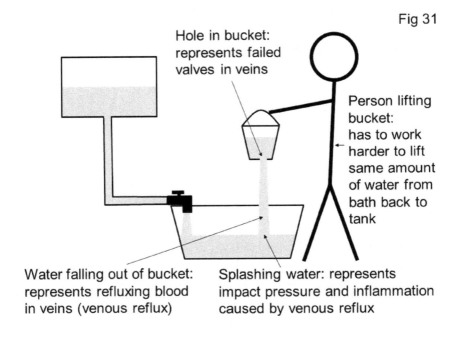

Fig 31

Hole in bucket: represents failed valves in veins

Person lifting bucket: has to work harder to lift same amount of water from bath back to tank

Water falling out of bucket: represents refluxing blood in veins (venous reflux)

Splashing water: represents impact pressure and inflammation caused by venous reflux

Figure 31: My "bucket" model to understand venous reflux. See text for details.

Now consider what would happen if you drilled a big hole in the bucket (Figure 31).

As the person lifts the bucket, some of the water starts falling out of the hole. As the person continues to lift the bucket more falls out.

It is clear that to empty the bath efficiently, the person is going to have to work harder and lift more buckets full of water to get the same effect, due to this hole. The bigger the hole is, the harder and faster the person is going to have to work. In addition, there may be more than one hole (Figure 32). This is frequently the case in venous disease where there may be in incompetent great saphenous vein but also several incompetent perforators.

Fig 32

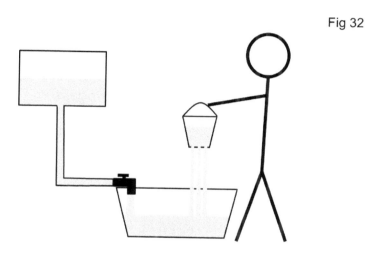

Figure 32: My "bucket" model to understand venous reflux. See text for details.

Because most people understand buckets, it is fairly obvious that if you were in this situation, you would fix the holes in the bucket. By saying "fix" you would understand that you would block off the holes. This would prevent water from falling out of the bucket.

In doing so, you will reduce the amount of work that the person has to do to keep the bath empty. The person will work less hard and less fast thanks to the fixed bucket.

If somebody asked you, "but where does the water go if you fix the holes?" you would probably think they were mad. You would naturally understand that by closing the holes, you have stopped water from falling out of the bucket when it is already being lifted back to the tank.

This is exactly the same argument as blood refluxing down an incompetent great saphenous vein, when it has already been pumped to the groin. The venous blood is already on the way back to the heart when it then falls back down the incompetent superficial vein. If you remove or block the vein at this point, the blood just continues back to the heart. If you don't, it falls down the vein and has to be pumped up all over again.

I hope that this helps you to understand why the treatment of venous reflux is to identify incompetent veins and to make sure that they are blocked off, preventing any reflux down them in the future. We are really just fixing the vein pump.

Now that we have understood this, we can go on to talk about which methods we can use to treat incompetent veins.

Chapter 9

Permanent treatment for venous reflux

The revolution in the management of venous leg ulcers should have happened in the 1990s, when it was discovered that most venous leg ulcers are caused by superficial venous reflux. As superficial venous reflux can be treated by using the same techniques that we use to treat varicose veins, we know that we can cure most venous leg ulcers. Of course, as noted before, this is dependent upon the patient walking and therefore getting the leg pump working again once we have fixed it.

For the rest of this chapter, we are going to discuss the treatment of superficial venous reflux. However, before we start on superficial venous reflux, we need to consider the much less common condition of deep venous reflux.

Deep venous reflux

As we have discussed in earlier chapters, venous reflux in the deep veins of the leg cannot be treated at the current time. Many doctors and nurses use this as a reason not to investigate patients with venous leg ulcers and consign them to dressings and compression treatment for the rest of their lives. However, as stated before, research has shown us that venous reflux in the deep veins alone, is rarely the cause of a venous leg ulcer.

As was first shown in the early 1990s, when patients with venous leg ulcers have a venous duplex ultrasound scan performed by a specialist vascular technologist or clinical vascular scientist in a specialist vein unit, it turns out that very few have reflux in the deep veins and most have reflux in the superficial veins. It also turns out that even if patients have reflux in the deep veins, most of the time this is associated with a blockage or narrowing that can be treated higher up. Or, they have superficial and deep vein reflux combined along with perforator vein reflux.

In both of these situations, the patient can now be improved with intervention, if not cured. In the first, the narrowing or obstruction of the deep veins that is causing the deep venous reflux, can be opened with a balloon and held open with a stent. In the second, it has been shown that treating the superficial and perforator vein reflux will improve the clinical situation, even although the deep venous reflux is left untreated.

Therefore, deep venous reflux is not the totally incurable problem we used to think that it was. Unfortunately, because this is not widely understood, many patients have been consigned to dressings and compression, and told that they do not have any other option, even though they have never had a venous duplex ultrasound scan performed by a specialist venous team.

So now we can turn to the much more common situation where patients have venous leg ulcers due to superficial venous reflux. This superficial reflux is usually in the great saphenous vein, small saphenous vein or in the incompetent perforator veins.

Superficial venous reflux and how to treat it

During my career in surgery, I have found that most surgeons have a conceptual problem when it comes to veins. If surgeons who treat veins have this problem, then it is not surprising that other doctors, nurses and virtually all patients have the same misunderstanding.

It appears that most surgeons, as well as most other doctors, nurses and members of the public, think that when you surgically remove something from the body, it has gone. They do not think about what the body might do as part of the healing process.

In one way, this is fully understandable. If for instance, a surgeon removes a gallbladder, then they know that the gallbladder has gone. They have cut through the skin, fat, veins and muscle to get to the gallbladder, which they have then removed. Then they sew all the layers back again. Over time, the patient recovers, and the body "heals".

However, let's just imagine that the surgeon has left something inside at the time of the original surgery. This is unlikely, but it helps us understand the argument. Let's think about what would happen if they must re-operate through the same area, one year later. In such a situation, the surgeon finds that when they cut through the healed wound, it bleeds profusely.

The surgeon must stop this bleeding as they cut through the scar. Of course, once they are inside, they find that the gallbladder has not grown back and is therefore not there anymore. Indeed, they would be very surprised if there was a gallbladder there. However, although they have encountered significant bleeding from the scar, they do not think about why the scar had bled.

However, thinking about this leads us to a quite startling realisation about veins. Generally, organs do not grow back. If you remove a kidney it is gone. If you remove a gallbladder or womb it is gone. You do not expect it to grow back.

On the other hand, when you have an operation, or damage yourself, you expect the skin, fat, muscle and other connective tissue to grow back again. This is called "healing".

Veins are part of the connective tissue. When they are cut or removed, they grow back. More importantly, not only do they grow back but when they grow back they have no valves in them. Therefore, when a vein grows back again after being damaged, as part of healing, it is always incompetent.

In varicose vein surgery, the surgeon aims to remove the target vein. However, just because a surgeon decides to remove a specific vein, it does not make that vein an organ. The vein does not suddenly change its nature and behave like an organ. It still behaves like connective tissue and will always try to regrow as part of the healing process.

It turns out that this concept is very important in the understanding of veins and the treatment of venous conditions. It is very important, not only in understanding how to cure venous leg ulcers, but also in how to stop varicose veins coming back again after treatment.

As we have seen in the last two chapters, the treatment of venous reflux disease is to remove or block off the vein. The traditional way of doing this has been to tie the vein, or to tie it and strip it away. We will discuss this next and show why it was such a bad idea.

Tying and stripping incompetent veins

Many people make the mistake of thinking that if you tie the top of an incompetent vein, it stops blood falling down into it (Figure 33). They seem to think the vein is like a bottle and when you put a cap on it, no fluid can get into it.

However, veins have lots of tributaries feeding blood into them. Therefore, although you might be able to tie the top of a vein, blood will still get into the vein through the tributaries. If the whole vein is incompetent, venous blood getting into the vein through the tributaries will still be able to reflux down the main vein, even though the top has been tied. Therefore, tying the top of the vein alone did not stop the venous reflux nor did it cure many of the problems caused by the venous reflux.

In the 1950s and 60s, some surgeons realised that just tying the top of the vein did not work and was associated with the venous problem recurring – usually varicose veins. Therefore, surgeons started tying the top of the vein and stripping the main section of the vein away in an attempt to stop the tributaries feeding blood into the incompetent vein (Figure 34). This was very painful and caused an awful lot of bruising. People having stripping were often given two weeks off work because of the pain.

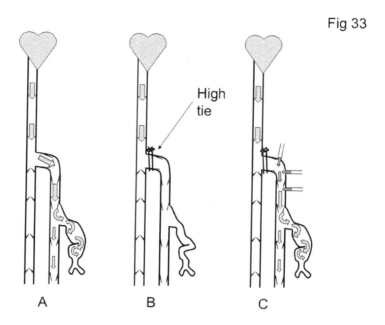

Fig 33

Figure 33: Diagram to show why the "high saphenous tie" ("high tie") didn't work for the treatment of varicose veins. Although traditionally it was thought that if you stopped blood getting into the top of the incompetent vein you would stop the venous reflux, experience showed that normal tributaries would still continue to empty blood into the great saphenous vein, and so reflux could continue.

However, it turned out that not only was this operation painful, but it frequently failed to work. The reason that stripping fails is that although the vein has been removed, the body tries to heal. Just as with any trauma, the body doesn't "know" that the surgeon wanted the vein gone. It just "knows" that the vein has been damaged and, as it is connective tissue, it tries to grow back (Figure 35).

Fig 34

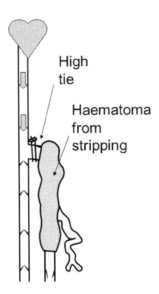

High
tie

Haematoma
from
stripping

Figure 34: Diagram showing what happened when the great saphenous vein was stripped out after performing a "high saphenous tie" – the classic "high tie and strip". In the short term, a large amount of blood collected in the tract of where the vein had been. This caused considerable pain and bruising.

Many surgeons find this very hard to believe – mainly because they don't want to believe it. As with many people, when surgeons learn how to do something from a person that they trust, they find it hard to believe that what they have been taught to do is wrong.

However, the fact that these veins do grow back, and grow back without valves, was proven by research that my team and I performed and have published. We showed this by following a group of patients who had undergone vein stripping in 1999 as part of another project. We followed this group of patients over many years, watching the veins grow back, using venous duplex ultrasound. The veins grew back through the bruising, becoming new incompetent varicose veins in exactly the same place that the original vein had been removed from. We published these papers in 2007 and 2015. Despite that, many doctors still perform vein stripping!

Fig 35

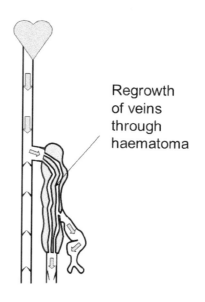

Regrowth
of veins
through
haematoma

Figure 35: Diagram showing the long-term problems with stripping the saphenous veins. Over months to years, the haematoma stimulated the normal healing process – and new veins grew through the area. These new veins ("neovascular tissue") would be regarded as normal healing if it occurred anywhere else in the body. However, in the leg, these new veins do not develop valves and so replace the incompetent vein that was stripped away with incompetent neovascular veins, which slowly dilate and cause the same problem to recur.

So, if tying the veins and stripping them doesn't work, what else can we do?

The next revolution in the treatment of varicose veins happened at the end of the 1990s when the new techniques of endovenous thermal ablation were developed. Although this may look like a complex name, it basically means that the veins were heated and destroyed from within. Let us look at this in more detail.

How to close a vein permanently - thrombosis versus fibrosis

Veins are tubes of living tissue. A vein wall is made up of protein, with living cells spaced throughout it (Figure 36).

Fig 36

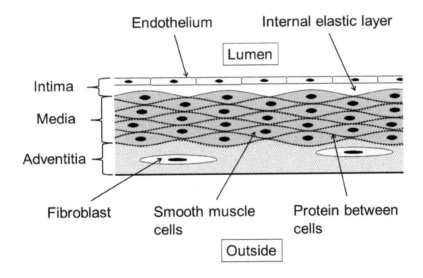

Figure 36: Diagrammatic representation of a vein wall. The three layers, intima, media and adventitia are shown, along with the specialised layer of cells that lines the inner lumen of every vein – the endothelium.

The vein wall has three layers. The innermost is called the intima. The middle is called the media. The outermost is called the adventitia.

To understand the next bit of how we cure ulcers by destroying incompetent veins, there are only a couple of things that you need to know.

Firstly, the inside of every vein has a single layer of cells called the endothelium. These endothelial cells line the insides of the veins like a pavement. They are very specialised and they stop the blood from clotting as it flows through the vein. If they are damaged, then the blood can clot within the vein.

The media is full of smooth muscle cells. These are the cells that can make the veins contract if you are cold and can let the vein dilate by relaxing if you are warm.

In the past, many doctors and nurses have thought that if you kill the endothelial cells using heat or sclerotherapy, then you can "stick" the wall together and this will "close" the vein permanently. Unfortunately, this does not happen. As many people know who have had sclerotherapy to veins in the past by people who do not understand the biological process, they can just come back again in the future. It is impossible to "stick the wall together" by damaging the endothelium alone.

It turns out that if you only damage the endothelium, you end up getting a clot in the vein called a thrombus (Figure 37). This thrombus is clotted blood and is full of stem cells. Because many other cells in the vein wall are still alive (particularly the smooth-muscle cells of the media) they work with the stem cells in the thrombus to heal the vein again. Slowly the thrombus reabsorbs, new endothelial cells grow onto the inner surface and the "closed" vein re-opens.

This is the reason why if you go into hospital and have a drip put into your arm, and then the drip stops working after a few days because the vein has clotted off, the next time you go into hospital you can almost always have the same vein used again for another drip. The clotted off vein has re-opened. This is also why many people get their varicose veins back again after treatment. Doctors who do not specialise in vein surgery frequently use the wrong treatment for the size of vein they are treating. Clot forms in the vein, a process called thrombosis. This then re-opens in the future, causing varicose veins to recur.

Conversely, if you kill the whole of the vein wall and don't leave any cells alive in it, and you can stop thrombus forming in the vein during this process, the vein wall will shrivel away to nothing, leaving just a tiny scar to show where it had been. This is a permanent closure of the vein and is called fibrosis (Figure 37). Once the vein has fibrosed, the body's immune system removes the fibrosed vein after several months, a process called "involution".

Fig 37

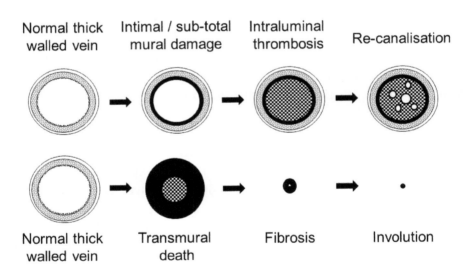

| Normal thick walled vein | Intimal / sub-total mural damage | Intraluminal thrombosis | Re-canalisation |

| Normal thick walled vein | Transmural death | Fibrosis | Involution |

Figure 37: Diagram showing the outcome of inadequate treatment, where only the endothelium and intima are damaged, resulting in "closure" by thrombosis only to re-canalise in the future, compared to transmural death as suggested by Mark Whiteley in 2004 which results in fibrosis and involution – a permanent "closure" of the vein.

In 1999, I realised that this was the mechanism that resulted in the successful, permanent closure of a treated vein. I published this idea in 2004 in a chapter of a medical book. I gave my idea the name "transmural vein wall death". It is this transmural vein wall death that we need to achieve when we treat an incompetent vein.

When we are successful at achieving this, we say that the vein has been "ablated". Many doctors who treat varicose veins still say that they can "close" the vein, but this doesn't really tell us whether it is a temporary closure with thrombosis which will only open up again, or a permanent closure by fibrosis. Ablation is always a permanent closure by fibrosis.

Endovenous thermal ablation - permanent "closure" of an incompetent vein

It is clear from what we have said so far, that to stop venous reflux in an incompetent vein, we need to completely destroy the vein wall and also keep thrombus (blood clot) out of the vein in the healing phase.

We can achieve this with endovenous thermal ablation.

Firstly, let's look at what we mean by endovenous thermal ablation.

The first word "endovenous" means inside the vein.

The second word "thermal" obviously means heat.

The third word "ablation" has been explained above.

Therefore, endovenous thermal ablation merely means permanently closing the vein by fibrosis, using heat from inside the vein.

The two most commonly used techniques to perform endovenous thermal ablation are either laser or radiofrequency. There has been some research using steam and microwaves, although these are not widely used at present.

In all endovenous thermal ablation techniques, a long thin tube called a "catheter" is passed into the incompetent vein under local anaesthetic. Ultrasound is used to get a needle into the vein, allowing a wire and dilator to be used to access the vein. Through this access, the catheter is passed up the vein, and is positioned precisely under ultrasound guidance.

Endovenous thermal ablation should always be performed under local anaesthetic to reduce the risk of deep vein thrombosis and nerve damage. Some doctors who are not confident at accessing the vein under ultrasound guidance, still use general anaesthetic to keep the patient still. However, this increases the risk of both deep vein thrombosis and nerve damage, and general anaesthetic is not needed. Nowadays local anaesthetic techniques are so sophisticated, patients should be able to walk-in, have the procedure, and walk out, without any sedation or additional anaesthesia.

The ultrasound is used to guide the device into the vein, and this is usually inserted around the knee or around the Achilles tendon. The device is then passed up inside the vein to the top of the section to be treated.

The patient is tipped head down, to drain all the blood out of the vein to be treated. By emptying the vein, we can ensure that all the heat produced by the endovenous device is used to ablate the vein. If there is any blood left in the vein, the heat is dissipated into the blood. This reduces the amount of heat reaching the vein wall, which reduces the chance of successful ablation. In addition, any blood caught in the vein and heated will form clot (thrombus) which further reduces the risk of successful ablation.

Fig 38

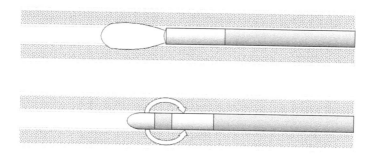

Figure 38: Diagram showing a jacket tip endovenous laser ablation device in a vein (upper image) and a bipolar radiofrequency ablation device in a similar vein (lower image). The laser ablates the vein by shooting energy forwards. The radiofrequency needs to be in contact with the vein wall as it passes an alternating current from one electrode to the other and back again. When this is done fast enough, heat is generated in the vein wall.

Therefore, it is essential that the patient is tipped quite severely head down at the point of treatment.

A lot of local anaesthetic called "tumescence" is injected around the vein containing the device. Again, this is injected under ultrasound guidance, to ensure that it is placed correctly around the vein that will be ablated with heat. This both makes it more comfortable for the patient during treatment and stops any heat transfer to healthy tissue when the vein is being permanently destroyed.

Depending on which technique is used, the vein is then heated (Figure 38) with enough energy to destroy the whole of the vein wall (Figure 39). The heat has two effects. The first is to shrink the protein in the vein wall, to physically close the vein and reduce the risk of any blood clot (thrombus) being left in the vein. The second is to kill all the cells in the vein wall, making sure that the vein will be removed bit by bit by the immune system, leaving only fibrosis and scar tissue. This disappears completely over 6 months to 1 year, and it is impossible for the vein to ever re-open again in the future.

Fig 39

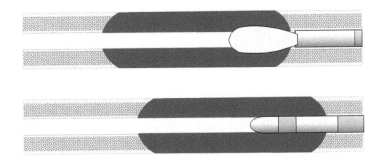

Figure 39: Diagram of the same two endovenous thermal ablation devices as in Figure 38, showing transmural ablation of the vein wall. This will result in a successful permanent ablation of the vein (see Figure 37).

Unfortunately, although this treatment is very easy in theory, in practice, many doctors find it difficult. Some doctors give too little power which only damages the inner wall of the vein (Figure 40). This results in the vein appearing to be closed on ultrasound because it is full of clot, only for the clot to dissolve over several

108

Fig 40

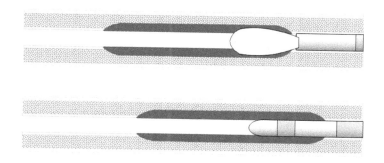

Figure 40: Diagram of the same two endovenous thermal ablation devices as in Figure 38, showing inadequate ablation of the vein wall, with only the endothelium and intima being ablated. This will result in an unsuccessful ablation of the vein with thrombosis and a high chance of re-canalisation (see Figure 37).

months and the problem vein to re-open in the future (Figure 37). Other doctors give too much power which can end up with charcoal being formed in the vein wall, and the vein bursting, causing a very painful recovery.

Over the last 15 years or so, my research group at The Whiteley Clinic has published and presented large amounts of research in this area. We have shown how to choose the optimal amount of thermal energy for veins of any particular size, to ensure the highest rate of ablation possible.

There are many different devices available, and different doctors will choose which ones they wish to use. The one that most doctors start with is the segmental radiofrequency ablation catheter as this is the simplest to use. It is basically just a long catheter with a section at the tip that gets hot. This tip is usually about 7cm long, but can range from 3 – 10 cm. When in position, the doctor just pushes a button and the device heats for a set treatment cycle. The doctor can then choose if more than one treatment cycle is needed, and the vein is treated in segments. This can be used for patients with simple patterns of venous reflux.

However, the problem with devices that have been "dumbed down" to be easy to use, is that they have certain defined settings and are not very versatile. These segmental devices cannot be used for short veins that are shorter than the heated tip, such as short sections of venous incompetence in previously treated veins that have re-opened, nor in incompetent perforators.

As such, more experienced doctors who deal with more complex cases tend to use devices such as laser, as these are more versatile. These devices have a very short tip, and doctors can choose exactly what power to use and how fast to pull the device through the vein to treat it. This allows both long sections as well as very short sections of vein to be treated successfully with the same device.

TRansLuminal Occlusion of incompetent Perforators (TRLOP)

Although most doctors and nurses have always concentrated on the two long veins in the leg, the great saphenous and the small saphenous veins as the source of venous reflux, research has shown that in ulcers, incompetent perforators are very important. Failure to treat the incompetent perforators may well mean that the ulcer does not heal, despite having had endovenous treatment of the long veins as above.

In 2001, Judy Holdstock and I developed the TRLOP procedure. TRLOP is simple, although technically demanding. With practice,

110

and good ultrasound, it is possible to successfully ablate 80-90% of incompetent perforator veins.

Very simply, an endovenous thermal ablation device such as a laser or short tipped radiofrequency device is passed into the incompetent perforator under ultrasound control (Figure 41). Local anaesthetic is injected around the vein, again under ultrasound control. A set amount of heat energy is passed into the perforator to completely ablate it using the same principles as above.

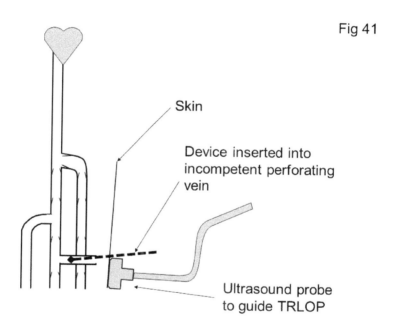

Fig 41

Skin

Device inserted into incompetent perforating vein

Ultrasound probe to guide TRLOP

Figure 41: Diagrammatic representation of the TRLOP (TRansLuminal Occlusion of Perforator) technique to ablate incompetent perforating veins. Invented by Mark Whiteley and Judy Holdstock in 2001, any ablation device can be used. Ultrasound is used to guide a cannula (tube) into the target perforating vein and the ablation device is passed along the dotted line in the diagram. Ablation – whether thermal or non-thermal – is then performed at the junction of the deep and superficial compartments (technically where the perforator perforates the deep fascia).

111

Non-thermal endovenous ablation

There are new techniques coming out which do not use heat to ablate the vein.

These non-thermal techniques are newer and have undergone less development than endovenous laser or endovenous radiofrequency. The two most commonly used are mechanochemical ablation (MOCA) or glue.

The technique of using them is very similar to the technique of endovenous thermal ablation. Ultrasound is used to place a catheter into a vein. The catheter is then passed up the vein to the top of the section to be treated. The advantages of these techniques are that they do not need the large volume of tumescent anaesthesia to be injected around the vein, as there is no heat generated in the vein during its destruction.

Therefore, as soon as the catheter is in place, the patient can be placed head down to empty blood out of the target vein and the technique started, without any more injection of local anaesthetic. This makes the procedure less uncomfortable for the patient. However, at the present time, both the MOCA and glue techniques are being assessed as to whether they get the same long-term outcomes that can be achieved with the endovenous thermal ablation.

Foam sclerotherapy

Sclerotherapy has been used as a method to ablate small veins for decades.

Sclerotherapy is performed by injecting a substance into a vein that kills the cells in the vein wall. The substance used is usually a detergent and the two most commonly used are called sodium tetradecyl sulphate or polidocanol. Both of these substances work by binding with the fat and proteins in the walls of the endothelial cells, and then pulling these sections out as the detergent also dissolves in the blood plasma. This process rips holes in the endothelial cells, killing them.

It used to be thought that by killing the endothelial cells, it would be possible to "stick the vein wall together". However, as we discussed above, this does not happen.

We have recently published research showing that when the endothelial cells die, they probably release substances into the vein wall that kills some of the nearby cells. This process is technically called apoptosis.

However, this effect only penetrates about 0.2 mm into the vein wall at best. Small veins have vein walls that are only about 0.1 mm, and therefore sclerotherapy can permanently kill these veins due to it causing transmural vein wall death.

Unfortunately, the bigger veins that cause venous leg ulcers such as the great and small saphenous veins, have vein walls which are nearer 0.5 mm thick. Hence, when these are treated with sclerotherapy, only the inner part of the vein wall dies, and the outer part of the vein wall is still living. As we have discussed above, this means that such treatment will result in some thrombus within the vein itself. As this thrombosis is reabsorbed, the vein is likely to re-open and venous reflux to recur again (Figure 42).

Another problem with sclerotherapy is that when liquid sclerotherapy is injected into a vein, it can mix with the blood itself rather than interact directly with the vein wall. As blood plasma is full of protein, and the blood cells have normal cell walls made up of protein and fat, the blood can bind with the sclerotherapy and inactivate it, before it destroys the vein wall.

To stop this from happening, in 1985 a man called Juan Cabrera patented a technique called foam sclerotherapy. He found that if the sclerotherapy is mixed with gas to make foam, and this foam is injected into the vein, then the foam will push the blood out of

Fig 42

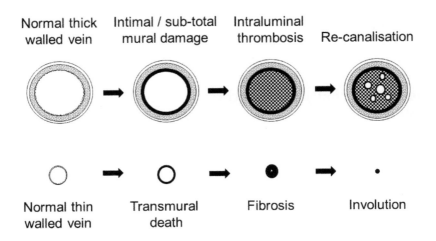

Figure 42: Diagram explaining why sclerotherapy works better in small veins than in large veins. As with thermal ablation, transmural death of the vein wall results in fibrosis and permanent ablation of the vein. Conversely, damage of the endothelium and inner layer of the vein alone results in thrombosis "closing" the vein, but with a high chance of re-canalisation in the future. Although most doctors measure the size of the vein, this makes it clear it is actually the thickness of the vein wall that determines success or failure of the ablation.

the vein allowing the sclerotherapy to interact directly with the vein wall (Figure 43).

The foam has a consistency very much like shaving foam and this technique has become very widespread in the venous world. Some doctors still use air to make their foam sclerotherapy, but this is regarded as sub-standard nowadays. Air contains nitrogen which doesn't dissolve well in the blood and hence bubbles can go to the brain and cause problems. Therefore, in the best vein clinics, either carbon dioxide or a mixture of carbon dioxide and oxygen is used as the gas when making foam sclerotherapy.

Fig 43

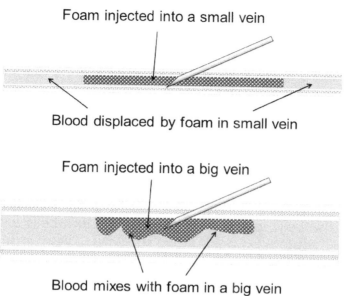

Foam injected into a small vein

Blood displaced by foam in small vein

Foam injected into a big vein

Blood mixes with foam in a big vein

Figure 43: Diagram showing that foam sclerotherapy displaces blood to get maximal contact with the vein wall. However, if the vein is too large, or the foam given too slowly or in too little amounts, it can mix with the blood. This will inactivate any sclerosant, and prevent it from acting on the target vein wall.

However, as discussed above, because sclerotherapy only has its effect up to about 0.2 mm into the vein wall, it is only really effective in small veins. Therefore, foam sclerotherapy is not particularly effective in the medium to long term when it is used by itself to treat the great or small saphenous veins, and the recurrence rates are high when compared with endovenous thermal ablation when used in these cases.

Because of our research, it has always been my practice to ablate the refluxing thick-walled veins with endovenous thermal ablation, and then come back a few weeks later to destroy the small veins and stasis veins with foam sclerotherapy. We have published our results to show that this approach permanently cures venous leg ulcers in 85% of our patients.

When foam sclerotherapy is used, it is important to understand how it works. It is not like cavity wall insulation where the foam solidifies and blocks the vein. On the contrary, the foam bubbles pop and the foam disappears within about 1 to 2 minutes of being injected. Once the foam has gone, the blood will be able to flow back into the treated section of vein.

If the endothelium has been successfully killed, any blood getting back into this section of vein will instantly clot on the dead cells and cause thrombosis. Not only can this thrombosis stimulate the vein to re-open due to the stem cells within the thrombosis, but thrombosis in a superficial vein is also very painful for the patient and can leave a brown stain on the skin. Therefore, good foam sclerotherapy is performed by injecting the foam and instantly compressing the vein with a bandage or stocking. This compression aims to keep as much blood out of the treated vein as possible. The compression should be left in place for 14 to 21 days to get the best results, as it takes this long for the dead vein to undergo fibrosis and be removed by the body's immune system.

This mechanism is different from endovenous thermal ablation where the vein shrinks during treatment due to the heat. As the vein shrinks there is no need for compression. In sclerotherapy, there is no shrinkage of the vein and therefore compression is mandatory for a good result.

Having looked at the treatment of venous reflux in detail, we are now going to see how venous stasis veins can be treated.

Chapter 10

Treatment of venous stasis veins

As we have previously discussed, blood stagnating in dilated veins under a venous leg ulcer or damaged skin in the lower leg, causes severe inflammation in the vein wall and surrounding tissue. This inflammation is due to the accumulation of carbon dioxide making the blood more acidic as well as the accumulation of waste products due to the blood cells staying alive.

Stasis veins can occur due to inactivity alone as we have previously pointed out. However, they are much more commonly found in association with venous reflux.

Many doctors who have treated venous reflux in patients with venous leg ulcers in the past, have seen an improvement in the venous leg ulcer but sometimes not a complete cure. It appears that one of the reasons for this is that it is not enough to take away the venous reflux and the inflammation associated with that, if you do not also take away the inflammation caused by the stagnant blood in the venous stasis veins.

Of course, anything that makes the blood less stagnant will help in the short term. Elevating the leg, movement or compressing the veins will get rid of some or all of the stagnant blood in the short term but will not cure the problem in the long term.

The venous stasis veins appear on ultrasound as a network of intercommunicating veins under the skin, but between skin and muscle. This is often called a "plexus". In many cases, the overlying skin is either broken down as a venous ulcer or is very hard and discoloured making any surgery virtually impossible.

Therefore, the ideal treatment for venous stasis veins is ultrasound guided foam sclerotherapy.

Using ultrasound, the network of venous stasis veins can be identified easily. Injections of foam sclerotherapy can then be injected into the stasis veins. Fortunately foam sclerotherapy can be seen clearly on ultrasound, as the bubbles appear white. Therefore, it is easy to follow the foam sclerotherapy and see which veins have been filled and which have not. In this way, several injections can be given to make sure that all of the venous stasis veins have been treated.

As we have described in the previous chapter, foam sclerotherapy works by pushing blood out of the vein allowing the sclerotherapy detergent to interact directly with the vein wall. This kills the endothelial cells on the inner lining of the vein wall, which then release certain substances that cause the inner 0.2 mm of the vein wall to die.

Fortunately, many of these stasis veins have walls that are only in the 0.2 mm range. Hence foam sclerotherapy is usually very effective at treating these networks of stasis veins.

Of course, as pointed out in the previous chapter, once injected the foam bubbles start to pop and the foam disappears. It is essential that blood does not get back into these dead veins. If it did, the resulting thrombosis would be very painful and would increase the risk of healing and re-opening of the veins. Therefore, as the foam sclerotherapy is injected, it is essential to bind the leg with a tight bandage.

This tight bandage should be left on for a minimum of 14 days and nights ideally and preferably 21 days and nights if possible. After 14 days and nights the dead vein wall should have completely fibrosed, permanently destroying and removing the vein. Therefore, when the compression is released, the vein will have shrivelled away and will be a fibrous mass of scar tissue. As the stasis veins will be ablated by the foam sclerotherapy, there will be no room for any stagnant blood and so there will be no further inflammation due to venous stasis.

Terminal Interruption of the Reflux Source (TIRS)

In 2010, a very innovative surgeon from the United States called Ron Bush described a new technique for treating venous leg ulcers cheaply and simply.

By 2010, it was well known by venous experts that most venous leg ulcers were due to venous reflux in superficial veins and associated stagnant blood in stasis veins under the ulcer. Many of us had been curing venous leg ulcers by endovenous ablation of the incompetent veins, TRLOP closure of the perforators and then a few weeks later destroying the stasis veins with ultrasound guided foam sclerotherapy. Indeed in 2013 we published our 12-year results of how successful this approach was.

However, Ron Bush came up with a different idea. In his technique which he termed "terminal interruption of the reflux source" or TIRS, the doctor ignores the venous reflux and just treats the stasis veins with ultrasound guided foam sclerotherapy. In this way, the inflammation due to the stagnation of the blood in the stasis veins is cured. In addition, although there is still venous reflux, any inflammation that is caused by the reflux is not transmitted to the area under the ulcer, because this has been ablated by the foam sclerotherapy.

It is a very good idea to get a short-term improvement or healing of a leg ulcer and is certainly worth considering in patients with painful leg ulcers who want a short-term boost. In addition, it is very much less expensive than doing the whole job and ablating the venous reflux first.

However, the concern is that if the venous reflux is not cured, it will obviously continue. This could mean that the chance of recurrent reflux, and hence recurrent ulceration, will be far higher than in those patients who have the venous reflux permanently ablated.

Now we have understood the treatment of stasis veins, we will look at how venous obstruction is treated.

Chapter 11

Treatment of venous obstruction

As we have alluded to in previous chapters, obstruction of the veins can either be a significant narrowing or blockage. Once again, we are not going to spend much time looking at this because obstruction accounts for a minority of venous leg ulcers. If patients with venous leg ulcers go through the proper investigations of venous duplex ultrasound scanning in specialist vein units, most will be cured by the treatment of venous reflux and stasis veins. Those that find they do have some form of obstruction will be identified, and a more in-depth conversation can be had with them at that time.

The commonest cause for a significant narrowing or blockage of the deep veins is chronic inflammation from previous deep vein thrombosis (DVT's) that have either been multiple or have lasted for a very long time. As with all chronic inflammation, this causes significant damage of the vein wall. This damage destroys the valves making the vein incompetent and causes scar tissue narrowing or blocking the whole of the vein. When this sort of damage occurs, it is called "post thrombotic syndrome" (PTS) (Figure 44).

Although we have said it before, it is worth reiterating that a single DVT that has been cleared quickly using anticoagulation, rarely causes this problem. This is very important because most doctors and nurses will always assume that a patient with a leg ulcer and the history of a previous DVT has got post thrombotic syndrome. As such they will probably not offer the patient a venous duplex ultrasound scan and will incorrectly tell the patient that they are incurable.

The poor patient will be told that they must have dressings and compression for the rest of their life. In most of these patients with a single DVT, the deep vein will actually be normal, and they would be fully curable using the techniques described in Chapters 9 and 10.

Fig 44

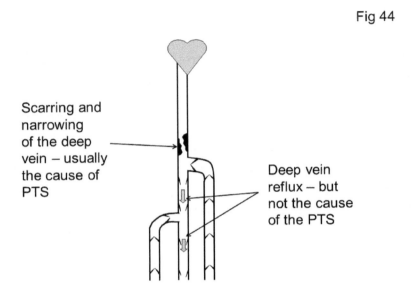

Scarring and narrowing of the deep vein – usually the cause of PTS

Deep vein reflux – but not the cause of the PTS

Figure 44: Diagram showing a common presentation of post thrombotic syndrome (PTS). Duplex shows reflux in the deep veins, but the actual problem is the obstruction in the pelvic veins due to scar tissue – not the deep vein reflux. This can be good news as such obstructions can often be opened up with a stent.

Another reason for narrowing or obstruction of veins in the pelvis is a condition called non-thrombotic iliac vein lesion (NIVL). In this condition, there is a narrowing on the inside of the vein in the pelvis. This is often very short and is often thought to be due to the remnants of a valve that should not be there. Quite often this cannot be found using duplex or MRI and is only seen with a very specialised test called intravascular ultrasound (IVUS). However, this is really quite specialist and not really a subject that we need to go into in great detail.

Sometimes, veins can be narrowed or obstructed due to structures on the outside of the vein pushing the vein shut. The most well-known of these (compression syndromes) is May-Thurner syndrome (Figure 21), where the artery in the pelvis crosses over the left pelvic vein compressing it. However, there can be other compression syndromes particularly behind the knee (popliteal compression syndrome).

In the past, treatment for venous obstruction used to be to perform a venous bypass operation. A typical operation would be to put a bypass (usually sew a bit of vein) from one groin to the other groin to bypass a blockage in the pelvis (Figure 45).

Nowadays, such bypasses are almost never needed. Modern technology has allowed the development of expandable stents that can be placed in veins and opened to keep the vein open.

A stent is a metal tube made from a latticework of fine metal that really looks like very small chicken wire. It can be introduced

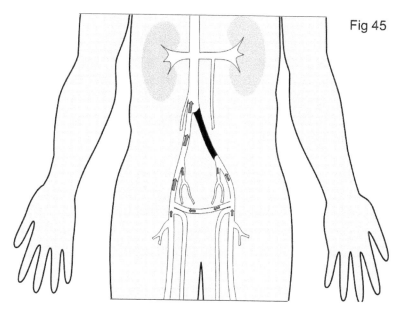

Fig 45

Figure 45: Diagram showing how a venous bypass used to be used to bypass a blocked iliac vein in the pelvis.

123

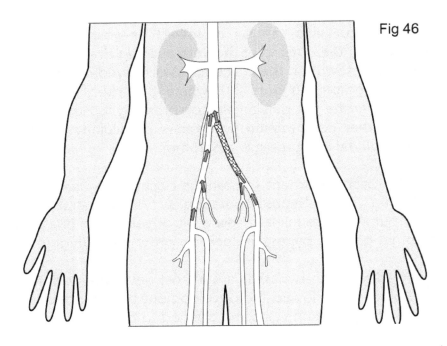

Fig 46

Figure 46: Diagram showing how this sort of blockage is treated nowadays with a stent.

into the vein through a single needle hole, usually in the groin. A wire is passed across the narrowing or blockage and in most systems, a balloon is then passed across the same section of vein. A balloon is used to dilate the narrowing or blockage and then the stent put in place and dilated to keep the obstructed section of vein open (Figure 46).

The ability to stent occluded veins has totally revolutionised the treatment of post thrombotic syndrome. Patients who have been told for years that they are untreatable and that they will have to wear compression to get any relief at all, are now getting near complete relief from their symptoms in many cases.

Once the obstruction has been relieved, any superficial venous reflux, perforator vein reflux or stasis veins can then be treated if necessary with the treatments in chapters 9 and 10.

If all patients with venous leg ulcers who could walk were referred to specialist vein units, the majority of such patients could have been cured if the investigations and treatments explained up to this point of the book had been followed.

Since July 2013 in the UK, the National Institute for Health and Care Excellence (NICE) has recommended all patients with venous leg ulcers to be referred and treated using these principles (NICE CG 168).

The next chapter will briefly look at the more traditional way of treating leg ulcers with dressings and compression.

Chapter 12

Dressings and compression for venous leg ulcers

Almost all "experts" in venous leg ulcer care still state that "compression is the mainstay of treatment of venous leg ulcers". This might be true because of the way that doctors and nurses have been taught, but if you have followed the information provided in this book to this point, you will realise that this is completely wrong.

If so-called "experts" keep quoting this out-dated mantra, then doctors, nurses, other healthcare professionals and even patients will just accept long-term compression and recurrent leg ulcers and will not set out thinking that venous leg ulcers are a curable condition in the majority of people.

The massive cost to the economy of failing to cure venous leg ulcers in terms of the huge amount of money spent on ulcer dressings, compression and nursing time could be cut to a fraction of the cost if the majority of patients with venous leg ulcers had the less expensive option of venous duplex scanning and curative treatment.

It is amazing that in a society that is meant to be cost conscious, governments and medical insurance companies try to put limits on surgical operations which could save them money. In the case of venous leg ulcers, funders of health care waste far more in the medium and long term by having to provide nursing and wound care than paying for a cure.

The arguments about quality-of-life of the patient and of their family and carers is self-evident.

Hence, the relegation of the discussion about dressings and compression to Chapter 12 of this book is deliberate, as this puts the importance of this part of the care of venous leg ulcers in the right priority with respect of what has been discussed before.

Without doubt, those patients who have been found to be incurable following a full venous duplex ultrasound scan in a specialised unit, or who are unable to be cured because they are immobile or too unwell to have local anaesthetic procedures, or who have complex leg ulcers that are not venous in nature, all need the full care of an expert in dressing and compression.

However, the majority of patients who currently have dressings and compression as their primary treatment would actually be curable if they were sent to a venous specialist team who performed a proper venous duplex ultrasound scan, and then treated the patient on the findings.

As such, the majority of patients with venous leg ulcers would not even need an expert opinion from a specialist in dressings and compression if they were referred properly in the first instance and were cured before the venous leg ulcer became a long-term problem.

Dressings for venous leg ulcers

There is a huge industry in producing different dressings for venous leg ulcers. There are vast numbers of dressings with many different properties that are sold to nurses and other healthcare professionals who dress ulcers. The market is huge in all Western countries.

Every so now and then one product becomes famous. For years people have talked about Manuka honey. However, neither manuka honey nor any other wound dressing actually makes much difference in terms of healing.

Proper reviews of the available research, such as the Cochrane database, which exclude studies that have been designed specifically to show the advantage of one sort of company's product, show that there is very little, if any, advantage to any ulcer dressing over any other. The most important point for any wound dressing is probably that it is comfortable for the patient.

However, there are a couple of principles that should be learnt and held close to the heart by anyone involved in leg ulcer care, whether it be someone who is treating them, or someone who suffers from them.

Firstly, no dressing has any effect at all on the stagnant blood in the venous stasis veins, the venous reflux nor the venous obstruction. Therefore, no dressing can actually have any real effect at all on the cause of a venous leg ulcer. Whether a dressing is nice to wear, smells nice, is comfortable, is absorbent, is bactericidal (kills bacteria on contact) or even helps skin cells grow back, it has no effect whatsoever on the underlying cause of the venous leg ulcer. As we have pointed out previously, if such an underlying cause is identified and treated, the leg ulcer will heal regardless of any dressing used!

Secondly, the very best ulcer dressing is nature's own. That is a scab. As discussed in earlier chapters, the body has its own ideal way of dressing any wound, including an ulcer. Plasma oozes out of the capillaries in the ulcer bed. If the ulcer is allowed to dry, the water evaporates leaving the protein behind. At first this is "mushy" and, with time, solidifies into a hard scab. All the germs are pushed away from the wound and, under the ulcer, the process of making a scab ensures a perfect environment for the tissue to heal. Under the scab, more plasma containing nutrition and growth hormones collects, helping the tissue to regenerate and the skin to regrow. Once the healing is complete, the scab will fall off.

The current nursing methods of removing scabs and allowing fluid to keep leaking out of ulcers not only ends up with maceration of the surrounding skin, often causing pain and an increase in ulcer size, but also ends up with the patient losing a considerable amount of protein.

Therefore, the use of dressings should be thought about carefully and the huge amount of literature that is produced on them should be considered only in the light of what we have looked at in this book. Studies of ulcer dressings that have included patients who have curable leg ulcers, will always appear to show good improvements with the dressing that has been used in that study.

Therefore, professionals should make sure that when they read a study, all the subjects used have had a full venous duplex ultrasound and any reversable cause for the ulceration has been treated before the patient is included. Patients should only be included in such studies if they have been shown to be incurable by venous intervention.

Compression for venous leg ulcers

As has been alluded to several times previously in this book, venous leg ulcers will always heal if you can remove the underlying chronic inflammation in the tissue and veins beneath the ulcers. After all, it is this inflammation that has caused the ulcers to form in the first place and is preventing them from healing permanently.

The easiest way to achieve this is to elevate the leg and to keep it elevated. As we have seen, this will empty the stasis veins, getting rid of the stagnant blood that causes inflammation, and also stops any venous reflux. In the rare cases of venous obstruction, elevation increases the venous pressure in the leg, helping the blood to flow through a narrowed segment, or around a blockage. Unfortunately, most people are not able to stay in bed with their leg elevated all day and so other ways to counteract the causes of venous leg ulceration are needed.

When a patient has to stand, sit or walk, they need to have

compression applied to their lower legs to reduce the chronic inflammation caused by the venous disease. As we have already stated, compression can help to resolve this inflammation in the following ways:

- Stagnation of blood in stasis veins - compression will compress the stasis veins, forcing the stagnant blood out of them and hence reducing the amount of inflammation in the veins and therefore also in the surrounding tissues

- Venous reflux - blood will always flow from an area of high pressure to an area of low pressure, accounting also for gravity. If compression is placed tightly around the lower leg, there is less of a pressure differential from the top of the leg to the bottom of the leg when compared to the same leg without any compression. Therefore, the speed and probably the amount of venous reflux is reduced and consequently so is the inflammation that it causes.

- Venous obstruction - in order to overcome any obstruction to flow, increasing the amount of pressure in the venous blood will help force more venous blood through any narrowing or, if completely blocked, through any natural bypasses. This reduces the amount of stagnant blood in the leg, once again reducing inflammation.

One of the consequences of inflammation is swelling. This swelling is due to fluid accumulating in the tissues. This fluid, when it is in the tissues, is called "oedema". Compression helps stop this fluid from forming, by pushing it back into the capillaries and small veins.

Therefore, it is clear that compression is beneficial in the short term, when applied to the legs of patients with venous leg ulcers. However, once you understand how compression works, it is also clear that compression has no long-term nor curative effect. As soon as the compression is removed, the original problem recurs, as compression only changes the underlying causes when it is applied. It has no benefit at all once it is removed. When compression is removed, the patient returns to the same state that they were in before the compression had been applied.

Therefore, despite huge amounts of research and volumes of books written on the subject, compression should be reserved for patients who are incurable, immobile or who cannot undergo venous surgery. The only other use of compression is to hold patients in as good a position as possible if they are waiting for surgery, or to compress veins following foam sclerotherapy or similar treatments.

Naturally, this will upset many doctors, nurses and other health care professionals who have been indoctrinated with the idea that compression is "all important" in the treatment and control of venous leg ulcers. However, as our own 12-year results have shown, as a treatment for venous leg ulcers, compression is only secondary to endovenous surgery, and most patients who are mobile will be able to do without it once their venous problems have been treated successfully.

Chapter 13

Summary and conclusions

I know that many will find this book shocking.

If that were not the case, there would be no point in me spending my time writing it, nor you spending your time reading it.

Many doctors, nurses and healthcare professionals involved in the care of patients with venous leg ulcers will find it shocking that their current standard of care is being questioned and that their continued dependence upon dressings and compression has been given such low priority. Those that feel this way, need to read the cases outlined in the cases section and need to follow the medico-legal case of the lady who is suing her doctors and nurses for not referring her as recommended by NICE Clinical Guidelines CG 168.

Much more importantly, any patients, families and carers will find it shocking that the people that they are trusting to look after their venous leg ulcers are not using knowledge obtained from research, that has been accumulating over the last two decades, to find a cure for this horrible chronic condition. They too will be shocked to read the cases that I have included to illustrate my position.

In 2011 I set up the Leg Ulcer Charity to try to educate patients, carers and professionals to know that most patients with venous leg ulcers are curable, and to empower patients to go out and ask why they are not getting the investigations and treatment that could potentially cure them. In some countries of the first world patients are already getting this. Unfortunately, in most they are not.

I am not sure that the Leg Ulcer Charity will survive as a charity, as it has not attracted a lot of support, and it might not be possible to continue it as a charity. However, whether it survives or not as an entity, I will continue to spread the message that most venous leg ulcers are curable, for the good of patients, their families and carers, the funders of healthcare (medical insurers or governments) and ultimately for the doctors and nurses who look after them. If only the doctors and nurses would adopt this approach and follow the current research and NICE guidelines, they would end up with more resources to look after those patients who are not easily curable.

I have tried to make this book simple and easy to read but, of course, like all areas of medicine, there is much more complexity hidden under every simple message. Despite this, the overall message of this book is correct.

To summarise the messages in this book

- Most venous leg ulcers are now curable, provided the patient is able to walk.
- All patients with a venous leg ulcer must have a venous duplex ultrasound scan.

- This scan needs to be performed by a specialist vascular technologist or clinical vascular scientist who specialises in venous duplex ultrasound scans, and who works as part of a specialist team including a venous surgeon.

- As there are few specialist venous surgeons, a vascular surgeon (a surgeon who specialises in arteries) may be part of the team, provided that they are experienced in venous treatments - especially endovenous surgery under local anaesthetic.

- Any superficial venous reflux should be ablated with endovenous surgery under local anaesthetic.

- Any incompetent perforators should be ablated by the TRLOP technique.

- Any stasis veins should be ablated by ultrasound guided foam sclerotherapy.

- Any venous obstruction in the pelvic veins should be stented if possible.

- Long-term compression should be reserved for patients who are found to be incurable having gone through the above assessments.

General messages

- Any patient with a venous leg ulcer has a high requirement for vitamin C and I recommend 1000 mg a day unless there is a contraindication to do so.

- Any patient with a venous leg ulcer requires a lot of protein and I recommend a high-protein diet.

- Any patient with a venous leg ulcer needs to stop blood stagnating in the lower leg. The best ways to stop this are walking, elevation of the leg, compression if the leg has to be down lower than the hip, stimulation of the veins by either external pump or a neuro muscular electrical shock causing a muscle twitch.

- Whenever possible, allow a leg ulcer to be exposed to the air. The air will kill any anaerobic organisms (bacteria that like to grow in conditions without oxygen), will allow a scab to form to create the perfect conditions for the ulcer to start healing and this will protect the surrounding skin from maceration.

- An ulcer with surrounding red skin which has shown microbes on a swab is not necessarily infected unless there are clear signs of infection as well. All ulcers will have some bacteria found on swabs as we are always covered with bacteria. Therefore, antibiotics should only be used if the patient is generally unwell or there is clearly an infection with spreading inflammation in the leg.